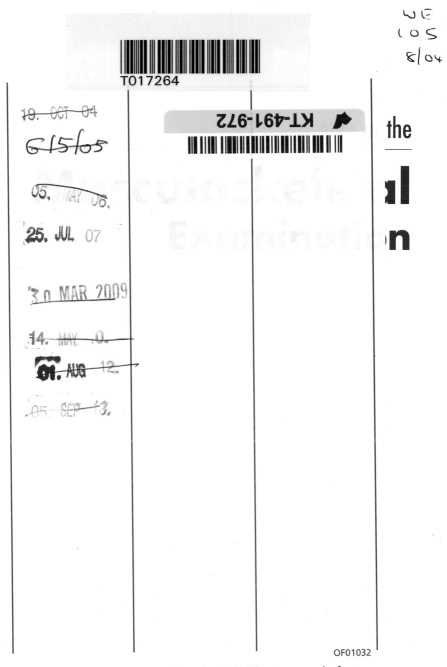

Salisbury District Hospital Library

Atlas of the
Musculoskeletal
Examination

Gerald Moore, MD
Professor, Section of Rheumatology
Department of Internal Medicine
University of Nebraska Medical Center
Omaha, Nebraska

AMERICAN COLLEGE OF PHYSICIANS
PHILADELPHIA

For a catalogue of publications available from ACP–ASIM, contact:

Customer Service Center
American College of Physicians–American Society of Internal Medicine
190 N. Independence Mall West
Philadelphia, PA 19106-1572
215-351-2600
800-523-1546, ext. 2600

Visit our Web site at www.acponline.org

Clinical Consultant: David R. Goldmann, MD
Acquisitions Editor: Mary K. Ruff
Manager, Book Publishing: David Myers
Developmental Editor: Alicia C. Dillihay
Production Supervisor: Allan S. Kleinberg
Cover and Interior Design: Colleen Ward/Fulcrum Data Services
Indexer: Nelle Garrecht

Manufactured in the United States of America
Composition by Fulcrum Data Services, Inc.
Printing/binding by Versa Press

American College of Physicians (ACP) became an imprint of the American College of Physicians—American Society of Internal Medicine in July 1998.

ISBN 1-930513-33-X

03 04 05 06 07 / 9 8 7 6 5 4 3 2 1

CONTENTS

INTRODUCTION: HOW TO USE THIS BOOK

Musculoskeletal problems or complaints are the leading cause of workplace illnesses and injuries in the United States and comprise the largest fraction of temporary and permanent disabilities (1). It is estimated that the cost of musculoskeletal care is in excess of $215 billion per year, with one in every seven Americans reporting some form of musculoskeletal complaint that limits activity or productivity (2). Although orthopaedists and orthopaedic surgeons are responsible for the majority of musculoskeletal care, a significant proportion of diagnosis and treatment is rendered by primary care physicians and other nonspecialist health care providers (3). Therefore it is imperative for the practicing physician to be prepared to undertake adequate examination methods that lead to effective treatment.

Atlas of the Musculoskeletal Examination, the first volume in the ACP Clinical Skills series, provides physicians with the most appropriate tests, concisely explaining what to look for and when to treat. General principles are initially discussed; subsequent chapters focus on the upper extremities (shoulder, elbow, wrist, hand/fingers), the spine and gait, and the lower extremities (hip, knee, ankle, foot/toes). Each test is accompanied by a photograph of the test being performed. Flowcharts provide the reader with an easy-to-follow guide to the particular examination being undertaken, with reference made to all appropriate illustrations. A selection of color plates appears at the end of the volume.

Range of motion is demonstrated for all joints, with specific examples given and potential problems noted. A few examples of specific disease processes are provided, especially when testing procedures are of value. Soft tissue diseases are very common causes of musculoskeletal problems and are emphasized where appropriate.

Excluded from this atlas are many of the specialized tests used primarily by orthopaedists. The physical examination of acute trauma of the extremities (e.g., examination for dislocation and fracture) has also been excluded. Pediatric disease processes are not emphasized. Description of these specific tests can be found in standard orthopaedic and pediatric textbooks. A focused neurologic examination should be performed when necessary, but here only selected neurologic tests are described.

The purpose of the author, therefore, and of the Clinical Skills series generally, has been to include those tests *most used and needed* by the primary care physician in his or her daily practice. Because of its conciseness and selectiveness, *Atlas of the Musculoskeletal Examination* is a work whose relatively short length ensures its frequent referral by the practicing health care provider.

GERALD MOORE, MD

REFERENCES

1. National Research Council and Institute of Medicine. Musculoskeletal Disorders and the Workplace: Low Back and Upper Extremities. Washington, DC: National Academy Press; 2001.
2. AAOS Bull. 1999;47:34-6. Also in Cooper JR. Musculoskeletal Conditions in the United States. The Medical Reporter. October 1999.
3. Musculoskeletal disease in the United States: who provides the care? Clin Orthop. 2001;385:52-6.

CHAPTER 1

GENERAL PRINCIPLES

Normal Examination

A complete musculoskeletal examination should be performed for all patients with complaints in and around their joints. If an abnormality is found in a particular joint, the opposite joint must be examined for symmetry. Any differences between the two sides usually suggest the possibility of major pathology.

An examination of the range of motion of the joints must be completed to determine the integrity of the joint. Active range of motion should be examined, if possible. This may be difficult in a patient with a neurologic deficit or severe pain, or in a patient who is uncooperative. In these situations, passive range of motion should be checked. Decreased range of motion suggests significant joint or soft tissue pathology (Table 1.1)

Table 1.1   Grading of Manual Muscle Testing

Numeric Grade	Descriptive Grade	Description
5	Normal	Complete range of motion against gravity with full or normal resistance
4	Good	Complete range of motion against gravity with some resistance
3	Fair	Complete range of motion against gravity
2	Poor	Complete range of motion with gravity eliminated
1	Trace	Muscle contraction, but no or very limited joint motion
0	Zero	No evidence of muscle function

From General orthopaedics. In: Greene WB, ed. Essentials of Musculoskeletal Care. Rosemont, IL: American Academy of Orthopaedic Surgeons. 2001:8; with permission.

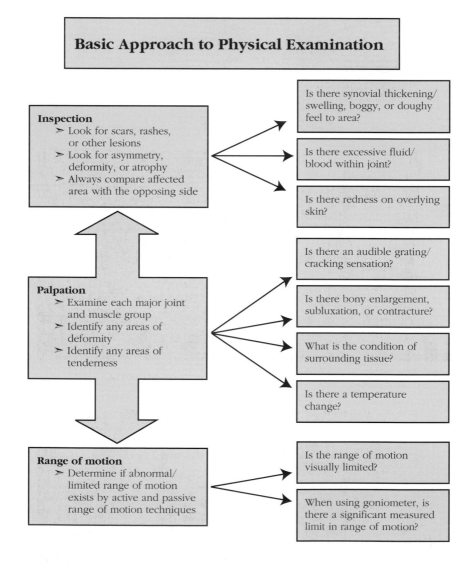

Basic Approach to Physical Examination

Inspection
- Look for scars, rashes, or other lesions
- Look for asymmetry, deformity, or atrophy
- Always compare affected area with the opposing side

Is there synovial thickening/ swelling, boggy, or doughy feel to area?

Is there excessive fluid/ blood within joint?

Is there redness on overlying skin?

Palpation
- Examine each major joint and muscle group
- Identify any areas of deformity
- Identify any areas of tenderness

Is there an audible grating/ cracking sensation?

Is there bony enlargement, subluxation, or contracture?

What is the condition of surrounding tissue?

Is there a temperature change?

Range of motion
- Determine if abnormal/ limited range of motion exists by active and passive range of motion techniques

Is the range of motion visually limited?

When using goniometer, is there a significant measured limit in range of motion?

FIGURES 1.1-1.3   Muscle strength. Decreased muscle strength may signify significant joint pathology, particularly when unilateral disease is demonstrated. Weakness around a joint can occur when pain from inflammation in the joint limits muscle function.

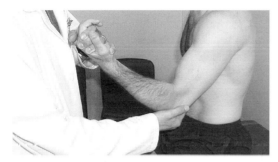

Figure 1.1 Testing muscle strength in upper extremity.

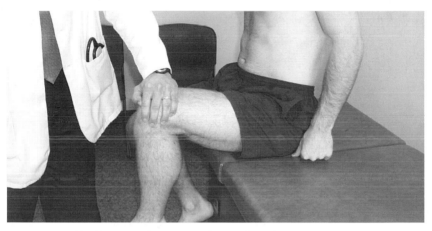

Figure 1.2 Testing muscle strength in proximal lower extremity.

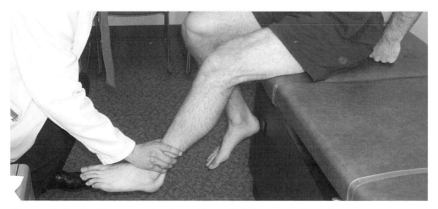

Figure 1.3 Testing muscle strength in distal lower extremity.

FIGURES 1.4-1.6   Concomitant neurologic examination. Primary neurologic disorders can sometimes be associated with apparent joint problems. A careful examination may distinguish between true joint pathology and complications of neurologic disorders.

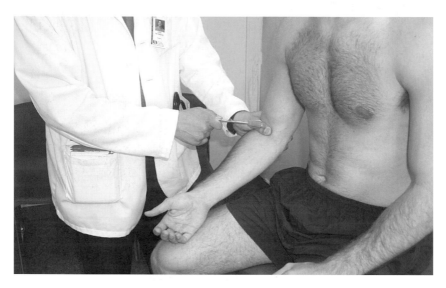

Figure 1.4   Testing for bicipital reflex.

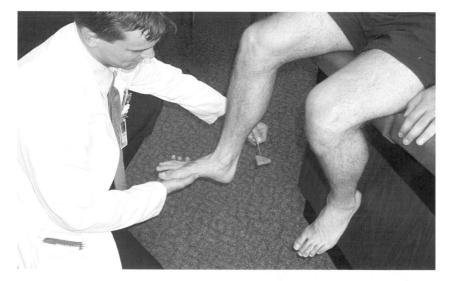

Figure 1.5   Testing for Achilles reflex.

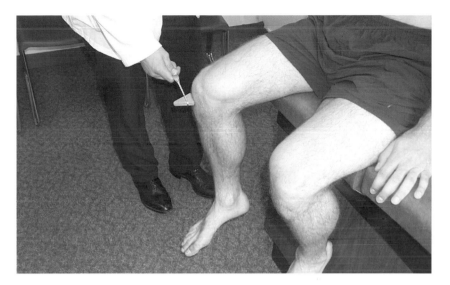

Figure 1.6 Testing for patellar reflex.

Abnormal Examination

Trauma

FIGURE **1.7** **Signs of trauma.** Examine the patient carefully for signs of trauma such as ecchymoses, swelling, and limitation of motion. Any unexplained findings must be thoroughly evaluated by taking further history, physical examination, and/or laboratory and radiographic studies.

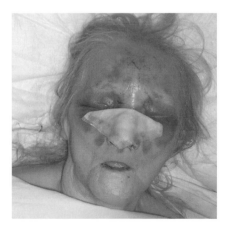

Figure 1.7 Patient with ecchmymoses secondary to head trauma (see Color Plate 1).

Inflammation

FIGURES 1.8-1.9 General signs of inflammation. Signs of inflammation (redness, swelling, tenderness, heat) occur with both soft tissue disease and joint problems. When present, inflammation may result from an infectious etiology, such as cellulites, or a systemic inflammatory process, such as rheumatoid arthritis.

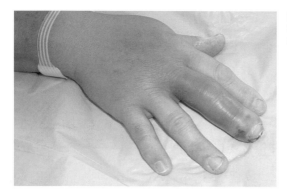

Figure 1.8 Osteomyelitis with cellulitis in third digit (see Color Plate 2).

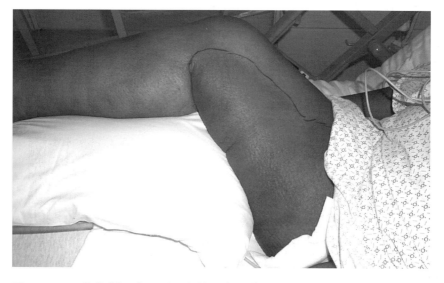

Figure 1.9 Cellulitis of proximal thigh (see Color Plate 3).

FIGURES 1.10-1.12   **Soft tissue involvement.** Soft tissue problems overlying a joint may be difficulty to differentiate from true joint abnormalities. Signs of inflammation should be sought. If the inflammatory response is not circumferential around the joint, soft tissue problems would be more likely. Soft tissue disease may limit range of motion in one direction but is unlikely to result in limitation at both extremes of motion.

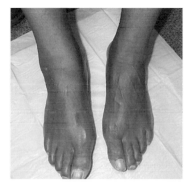

Figure 1.10   Inflammation of right ankle (see Color Plate 4).

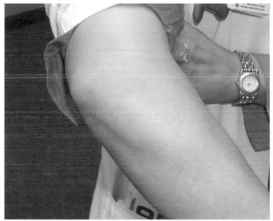

Figure 1.11   Cellulitis of elbow (see Color Plate 5).

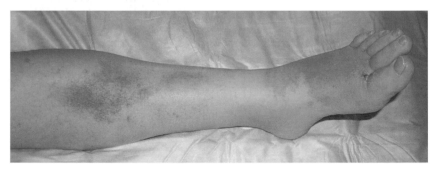

Figure 1.12   Cellulitis of lower leg (see Color Plate 6).

FIGURES 1.13-1.14   Joint disease. Arthritis may present with pain, signs of inflammation, joint effusion, instability, or other problems. A thorough examination can help to identify underlying pathology and determine appropriate therapy. Bony enlargement may be a manifestation of previous joint damage.

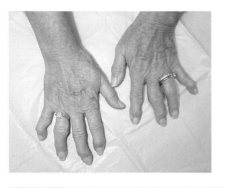

Figure 1.13 Degenerative arthritis in fingers.

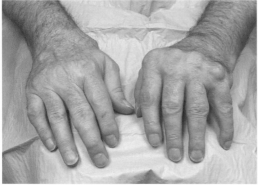

Figure 1.14 Deforming rheumatoid arthritis of hand.

CHAPTER 2

UPPER EXTREMITIES

Joint and soft tissue complaints of the upper extremities can cause significant disability from pain, decreased range of motion, or inability to perform the tasks of daily living. Complete examination of the involved areas is necessary to determine the cause of the patient's problems and develop an appropriate treatment plan.

Shoulder

FIGURES 2.1-2.8 Motions of the shoulder. Range of motion of the shoulder is decreased by many injuries and soft tissue complaints. Six different motions of the joint should be examined: flexion, extension, abduction, adduction, internal, and external rotation. Forward flexion goes to 180° with 60° of extension. Abduction is normally 180° with 50° of adduction. Ninety degrees of both internal and external rotation should be present. The elbow should be flexed to 90° while the shoulder is either in the neutral position or abducted to 90°.

Figure 2.1 Shoulder flexion.

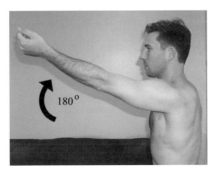

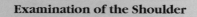

Examination of the Shoulder

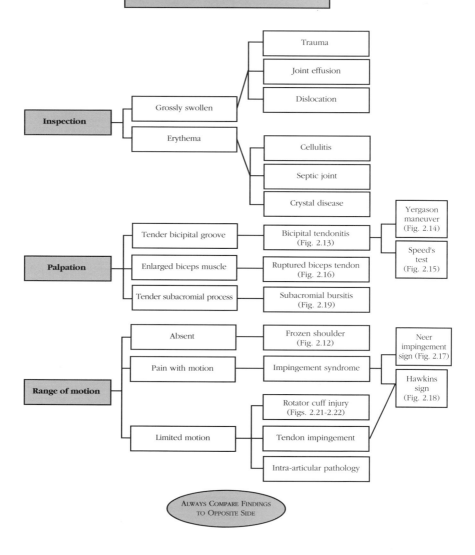

Always Compare Findings to Opposite Side

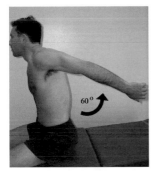

Figure 2.2 Shoulder extension.

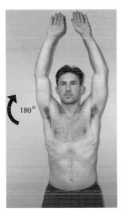

Figure 2.3 Shoulder abduction.

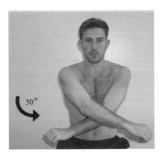

Figure 2.4 Shoulder adduction.

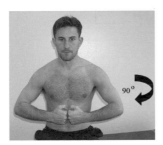

Figure 2.5 Internal rotation (shoulder in neutral position).

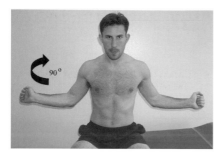

Figure 2.6 External rotation (shoulder in neutral position).

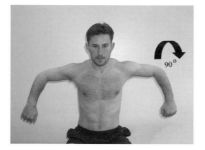

Figure 2.7 Internal rotation (shoulder abducted).

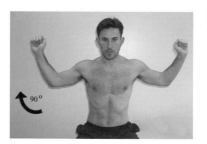

Figure 2.8 External rotation (shoulder abducted).

FIGURES 2.9-2.10 **"Scratch" test.** The "scratch" test combines all motions of the shoulder and is an easy way to screen for decreased range of motion.

Figure 2.9 "Scratch" test with arm above shoulder joint.

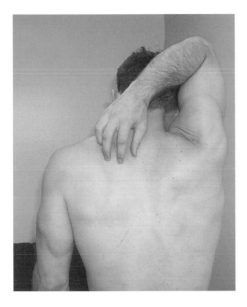

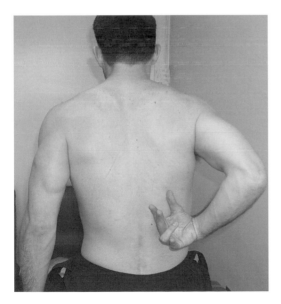

Figure 2.10 "Scratch" test with arm below shoulder joint.

FIGURE 2.11 **Passive range of motion.** Passive range of motion should be checked if the active range of motion is decreased. Place one hand on the shoulder and feel for the scapular spine. Motion of the scapula before 90° suggests shoulder pathology. Common causes of decreased range of motion of the shoulder include dislocation, tendonitis, rotator cuff injury, and joint pathology.

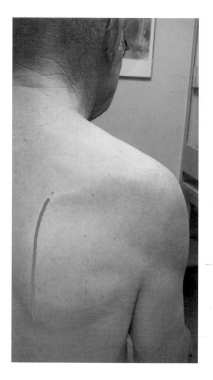

Figure 2.11 Shoulder in neutral position with spine of scapula identified.

FIGURE 2.12   **Frozen shoulder.** A major decrease in the range of motion of the shoulder is characteristic of a frozen shoulder. This is the end result of major soft tissue or bony trauma to the shoulder. Active range of motion is significantly decreased. Scapular motion before the shoulder is abducted to 90° is commonly found.

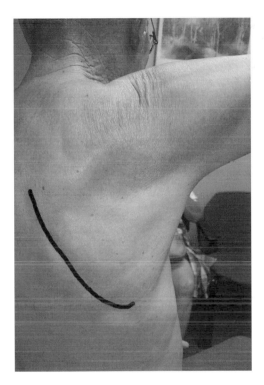

Figure 2.12   Frozen shoulder. Noticeable movement of scapula before 90°.

FIGURE 2.13   **Bicipital tendonitis.** Tenderness over the bicipital groove is typically found in bicipital tendonitis. The groove is located on the head of the humerus lateral to the coracoid process. Impingement of the bicipital tendon by the acromion is thought to be the etiology in many cases.

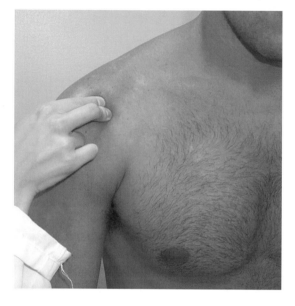

Figure 2.13   Palpation of bicipital groove.

FIGURE 2.14   **Yergason maneuver.** The Yergason maneuver is used to confirm the diagnosis of bicipital tendonitis. With the elbow flexed at 90° and the forearm pronated, the patient is asked to grasp two fingers of the examiner's hand. The patient should supinate the forearm against resistance by the examiner's fingers. Patients with tendonitis will complain of pain in the area of the bicipital groove.

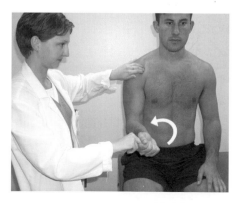

Figure 2.14   Yergason maneuver for bicipital tendonitis.

FIGURE **2.15** **Speed's test.** Forward flexion of the arm with the palm upward is performed against the resistance of the examiner's arm. Pain in the biciptal groove will occur with tendonitis.

Figure 2.15 Speed's test.

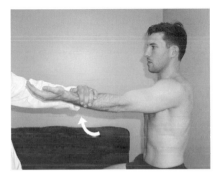

FIGURE **2.16** **Ruptured biceps tendon.** Swelling of the forearm in the area of the biceps muscle is characteristic of a ruptured bicipital tendon. In most cases this is asymptomatic and requires no specific treatment. Younger individuals may require surgical repair.

Figure 2.16 Ruptured bicipital tendon.

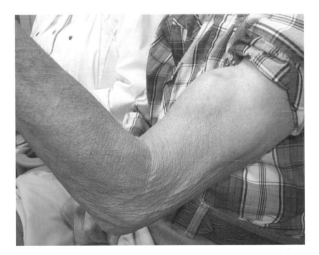

Impingement Syndrome (Rotator Cuff Tendonitis)

Impingement of any of the soft tissue structures of the shoulder can result in pain and decreased active range of motion. Pain is usually much decreased when passive range of motion is checked.

FIGURE 2.17 Neer impingement sign. Actively flexing and internally rotating the shoulder while stabilizing the scapula demonstrate the Neer impingement sign. Pain in the region of the subacromial bursa is found and is relieved by injection of an anesthetic into the bursa.

Figure 2.17 Neer impingement sign.

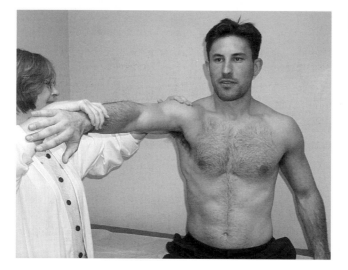

FIGURE 2.18 **Hawkins impingement sign.** The Hawkins impingement sign is performed by having the patient abduct and internally rotate the shoulder while the scapula is stabilized. Pain in the region of the subacromial bursa is found and is relieved by an injection of an anesthetic into the bursa.

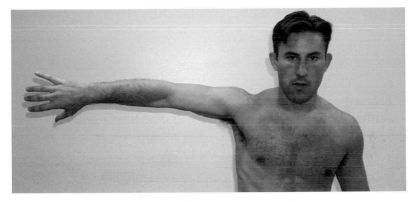

Figure 2.18 Hawkins impingement sign.

FIGURE 2.19 **Subacromial bursitis.** Inflammation of the subacromial bursa causes pain in the lateral aspect of the shoulder. The patient will complain of significant pain with abduction (particularly greater than 90°). Passive range of motion will cause much less pain. The impingement signs (Figures 2.17 and 2.18) will be positive.

Figure 2.19 Location of subacromial bursa.

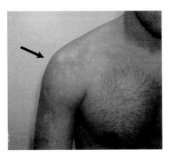

FIGURE 2.20 **Sulcus sign.** The patient is placed in a sitting position while the arm is pulled inferiorly. Patients with inferior glenohumeral instability will develop a "groove" in the acromiohumeral sulcus.

Figure 2.20 Sulcus sign.

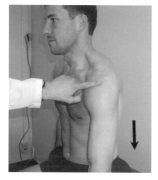

FIGURES 2.21-2.22 **Rotator cuff injury.** The rotator cuff stabilizes the shoulder as well as initiates abduction. It is composed of the subscapularis, infraspinatus, teres minor, and supraspinatus muscles. Injury to this structure is associated with significant limitation of motion, pain, and swelling. After an acute injury, it is difficult to examine the rotator cuff adequately because of inflammation. After a period of several weeks to months, the primary finding on physical examination will be that of a complete or partial frozen shoulder.

Figure 2.21 Rotator cuff: anterior view.

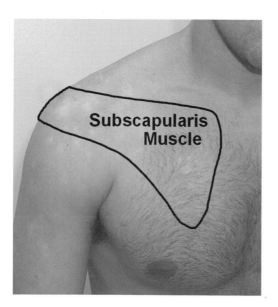

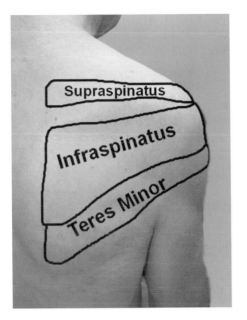

Figure 2.22 Rotator cuff: posterior view.

Elbow

FIGURES 2.23-2.25   General examination of the elbow. The elbow is a hinge joint formed by the humerus, radius, and ulna. Normal range of motion is flexion to 160° and extension to 0°. Females may demonstrate extension to −10 or −15°. The patient should supinate and pronate the forearm with the elbow flexed to 90°. Significant limitation of supination suggests disease of the radial head.

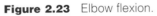

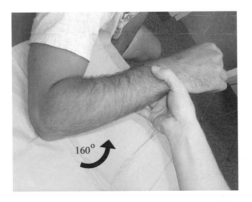

Figure 2.23 Elbow flexion.

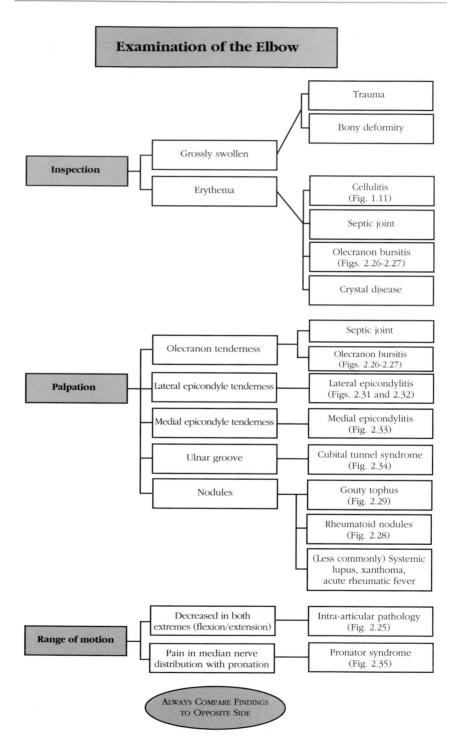

Examination of the Elbow

Inspection
- Grossly swollen
  - Trauma
  - Bony deformity
- Erythema
  - Cellulitis (Fig. 1.11)
  - Septic joint
  - Olecranon bursitis (Figs. 2.26-2.27)
  - Crystal disease

Palpation
- Olecranon tenderness
  - Septic joint
  - Olecranon bursitis (Figs. 2.26-2.27)
- Lateral epicondyle tenderness
  - Lateral epicondylitis (Figs. 2.31 and 2.32)
- Medial epicondyle tenderness
  - Medial epicondylitis (Fig. 2.33)
- Ulnar groove
  - Cubital tunnel syndrome (Fig. 2.34)
- Nodules
  - Gouty tophus (Fig. 2.29)
  - Rheumatoid nodules (Fig. 2.28)
  - (Less commonly) Systemic lupus, xanthoma, acute rheumatic fever

Range of motion
- Decreased in both extremes (flexion/extension)
  - Intra-articular pathology (Fig. 2.25)
- Pain in median nerve distribution with pronation
  - Pronator syndrome (Fig. 2.35)

ALWAYS COMPARE FINDINGS TO OPPOSITE SIDE

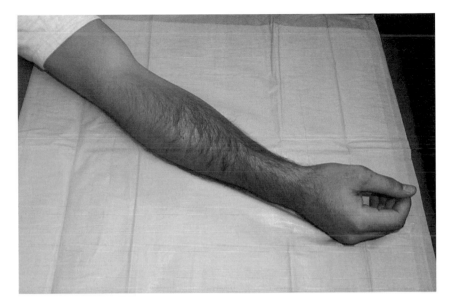

Figure 2.24 Elbow extension.

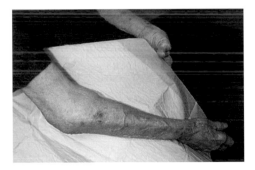

Figure 2.25 Limited extension and supination in patient with rheumatoid arthritis.

FIGURES 2.26-2.27 **Olecranon bursitis.** Swelling of the area around the elbow may be associated with olecranon bursitis or nodules of the extensor surface, or may be indicative of arthritis. The olecranon bursa may become inflamed secondary to an infectious agent or due to chronic irritation. Palpation of the area will reveal swelling with or without tenderness. Erythema and heat in the area are suggestive of an infected bursa (*Staphylococcus aureus* is commonly found). Limitation of motion is generally not a significant problem.

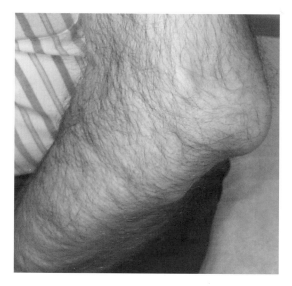

Figure 2.26 Noninflamed olecranon bursa.

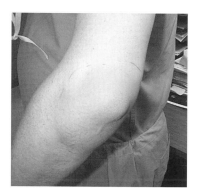

Figure 2.27 Inflamed olecranon bursa (see Color Plate 7).

FIGURES 2.28-2.29 **Subcutaneous nodules.** Fixed or moveable nodules on the extensor surfaces of the elbow may be seen with gout or rheumatoid arthritis. The nodules may be smooth or irregular in shape. Differentiation between gout and rheumatoid arthritis is difficult and requires a complete musculoskeletal examination to identify the source of the nodules. Other, less common, causes of nodules at the elbow include xanthoma, systemic lupus erythematosus, and acute rheumatic fever.

Figure 2.28 Nodule on extensor surface of forearm.

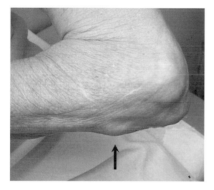

Figure 2.29 Gouty tophus of elbow.

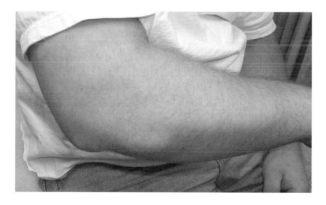

FIGURE 2.30   Synovitis of the elbow. Synovitis of the elbow joint is best determined through palpation of the ulnar groove. Place your finger longitudinally in the ulnar groove and attempt to displace the finger either medially or laterally. In the normal thin individual, the finger cannot be moved in either direction. The radial groove is not as prominent and therefore not easily palpated.

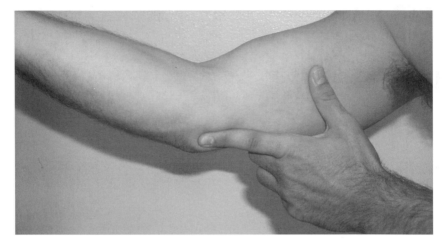

Figure 2.30   Palpation of ulnar groove.

Epicondylitis

FIGURES 2.31-2.32   Lateral epicondylitis. Commonly known as *tennis elbow,* lateral epicondylitis is a frequent cause of elbow pain. The patient may complain of diffuse elbow pain that, upon examination, is localized to the area of the lateral epicondyle. Maximum pain generally occurs at a point 1 to 2 cm distal to the lateral epicondyle. Active dorsiflexion of the wrist against resistance will reproduce the pain.

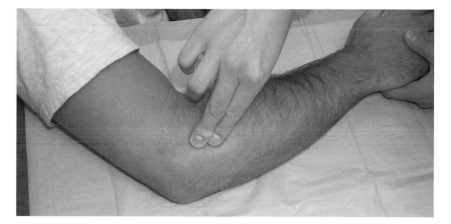

Figure 2.31 Palpation of lateral epicondyle.

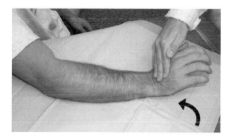

Figure 2.32 Stress test for lateral epicondylitis.

FIGURE 2.33 Medial epicondylitis. Medial epicondylitis is an overuse syndrome associated with pain over the medial epicondyle of the elbow. Palpation in the area will reproduce the pain.

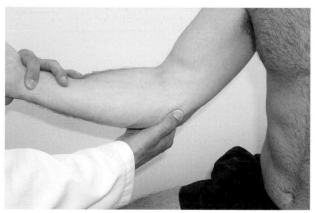

Figure 2.33
Palpation of medial epicondyle.

FIGURE 2.34 **Ulnar nerve entrapment (cubital tunnel syndrome).** The ulnar nerve is compressed at the elbow by the flexor carpi ulnaris muscle resulting in symptoms of numbness and tingling in the ring and little finger. Palpation of the ulnar groove may aggravate the ulnar nerve compression.

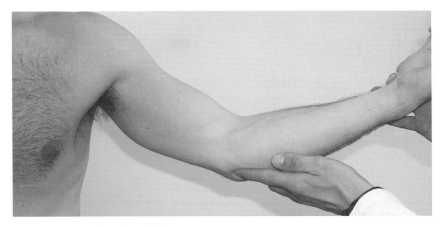

Figure 2.34 Palpation of ulnar groove.

FIGURE 2.35 **Pronator syndrome.** Occasionally, the pronator teres muscle can cause impingement on the median nerve in the upper forearm. Ask if the patient feels pain when pronating the forearm against resistance.

Figure 2.35 Test for pronator syndrome.

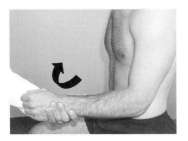

Wrist

FIGURES 2.36-2.39 General examination of the wrist. Wrist range of motion is complex. The patient should be able to palmar flex to 90° and dorsiflex to 70°. Ulnar deviation is approximately 50°, and radial deviation will be 20 to 30° in the normal individual.

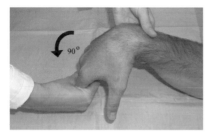

Figure 2.36 Wrist flexion.

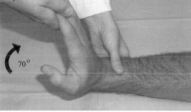

Figure 2.37 Wrist extension.

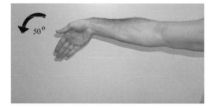

Figure 2.38 Ulnar deviation of wrist.

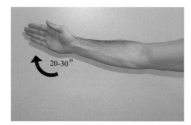

Figure 2.39 Radial deviation of wrist.

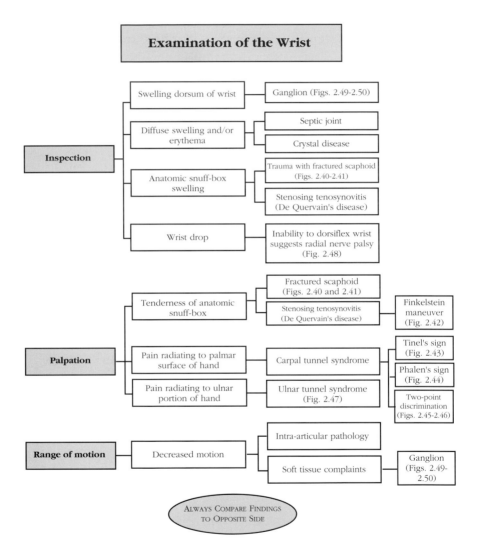

Examination of the Wrist

Inspection

Swelling dorsum of wrist — Ganglion (Figs. 2.49-2.50)

Diffuse swelling and/or erythema
- Septic joint
- Crystal disease

Anatomic snuff-box swelling
- Trauma with fractured scaphoid (Figs. 2.40-2.41)
- Stenosing tenosynovitis (De Quervain's disease)

Wrist drop — Inability to dorsiflex wrist suggests radial nerve palsy (Fig. 2.48)

Palpation

Tenderness of anatomic snuff-box
- Fractured scaphoid (Figs. 2.40 and 2.41)
- Stenosing tenosynovitis (De Quervain's disease) — Finkelstein maneuver (Fig. 2.42)

Pain radiating to palmar surface of hand — Carpal tunnel syndrome
- Tinel's sign (Fig. 2.43)
- Phalen's sign (Fig. 2.44)

Pain radiating to ulnar portion of hand — Ulnar tunnel syndrome (Fig. 2.47) — Two-point discrimination (Figs. 2.45-2.46)

Range of motion

Decreased motion
- Intra-articular pathology
- Soft tissue complaints — Ganglion (Figs. 2.49-2.50)

ALWAYS COMPARE FINDINGS TO OPPOSITE SIDE

Scaphoid Fracture and Stenosing Tenosynovitis

Acute pain in the snuff-box should suggest two primary diagnoses: scaphoid fracture or stenosing tenosynovitis (De Quervain's disease).

FIGURES 2.40-2.41   Scaphoid fracture. If acute trauma has occurred, consider the possibility of a fracture of the scaphoid. Initial radiographs may be normal. The patient should always be treated as if a fracture were present and x-rayed again one week later to see if a fracture has become visible.

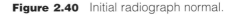

Figure 2.40   Initial radiograph normal.

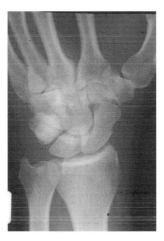

Figure 2.41   Follow-up radiograph one week later showing fracture line.

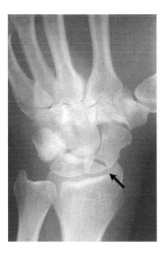

FIGURE 2.42   **Stenosing tenosynovitis (De Quervain's disease).** Stenosing tenosynovitis is an inflammation of the abductor pollicis longus and extensor pollicis brevis tendons. In the Finkelstein maneuver, the patient is asked to place his thumb in his palm and make a fist with ulnar deviation of the hand. Patients with stenosing tenosynovitis will have severe pain in the area of the tendon sheaths.

Figure 2.42   Finkelstein maneuver.

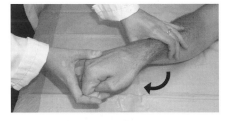

Carpal Tunnel Syndrome

A common cause of hand pain is carpal tunnel syndrome (compression of the median nerve at the wrist by the flexor retinaculum). The patient complains of pain in the hand (classically in the palm and palmar surface of the first three and a half digits). The patient may give the classic history of awakening at night with numbness in the hand, which causes him to shake the hand to decrease the symptoms. The patient may also give a history of pain while driving or during activities requiring him to hold his hands in the air.

FIGURE 2.43   **Tinel's sign.** Tapping lightly on the median nerve distal to the distal wrist crease will duplicate the patient's symptoms if carpal tunnel is present.

Figure 2.43
Tinel's sign.

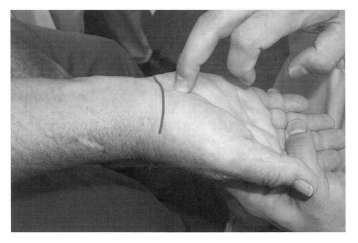

FIGURE 2.44 **Phalen's sign.** An alternative method of checking for carpal tunnel syndrome is to ask the patient to oppose the dorsum of both hands together and hold that position for 30 to 60 seconds. Numbness and tingling in the distribution of the median nerve is a positive sign.

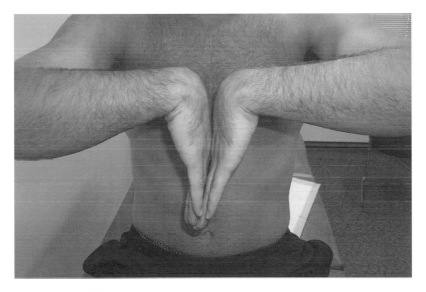

Figure 2.44 Phalen's sign.

FIGURES 2.45-2.46 Two-point discrimination. Patients with carpal tunnel syndrome will demonstrate decreased two-point discrimination of the hand. Normally, a patient will be able to discriminate sharp objects as close as 6 mm apart.

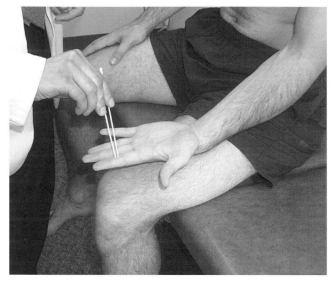

Figure 2.45
Checking for close discrimination.

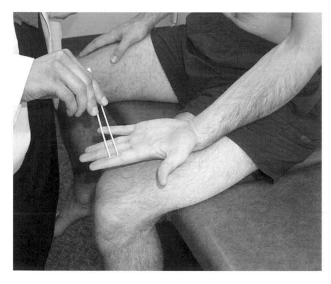

Figure 2.46
Checking for wider discrimination.

FIGURE 2.47 **Ulnar tunnel syndrome.** The ulnar nerve is compressed in Guyon's canal between the pisiform and the hook of the hamate. Symptoms of ulnar neuropathy will be present (see Figure 2.34).

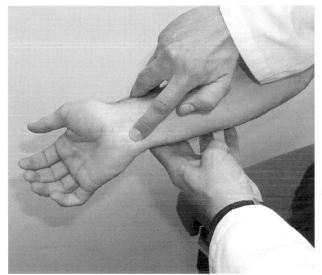

Figure 2.47
Location of Guyon's canal.

FIGURE 2.48 **Radial nerve palsy.** The radial nerve may be compressed in the spiral groove of the humerus, resulting in wrist drop, flexion of the metacarpal phalangeal joints, and adduction of the thumb. "Saturday night palsy", compression of the radial nerve when hanging the arm over the back of a chair, is another cause of wrist drop. Weakness of muscles supplied by the radial nerve may occur (brachioradialis and triceps muscles).

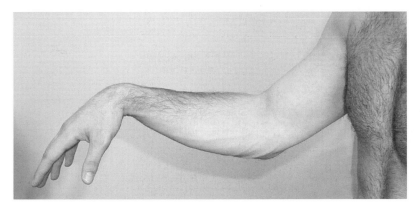

Figure 2.48 Demonstration of wrist drop.

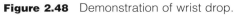

FIGURES 2.49-2.50   Ganglion. A ganglion is a synovial cyst of the wrist that manifests as a painless swelling on the dorsum of the wrist. However, ganglia can be demonstrated on the palmar surface as well. Palpation will reveal a smooth, fixed cystic structure. Limitation of wrist motion may be found in some individuals. Treatment is usually not necessary, because the ganglion will spontaneously regress in a few weeks to months. If surgical therapy is required, a complete synovectomy of the wrist is commonly performed.

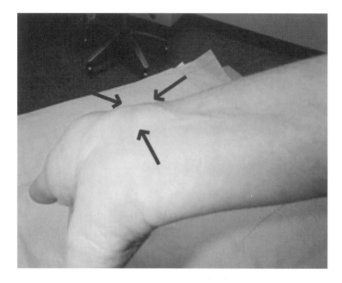

Figure 2.49
Ganglion on palmar surface of wrist.

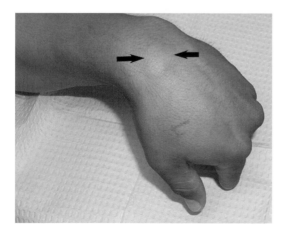

Figure 2.50   Ganglion on dorsal surface of wrist.

Hand and Fingers

FIGURES 2.51-2.52 **General examination of hand and fingers.** Numerous soft tissue and joint abnormalities can be seen in the fingers. Ask the patient to extend and spread his fingers and then make a fist to check for range of motion. Palpation of the joints should be done in a bimanual fashion.

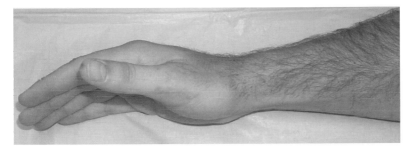

Figure 2.51 Range of motion of fingers: extension.

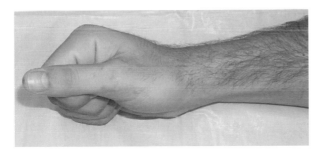

Figure 2.52 Range of motion of fingers: fist.

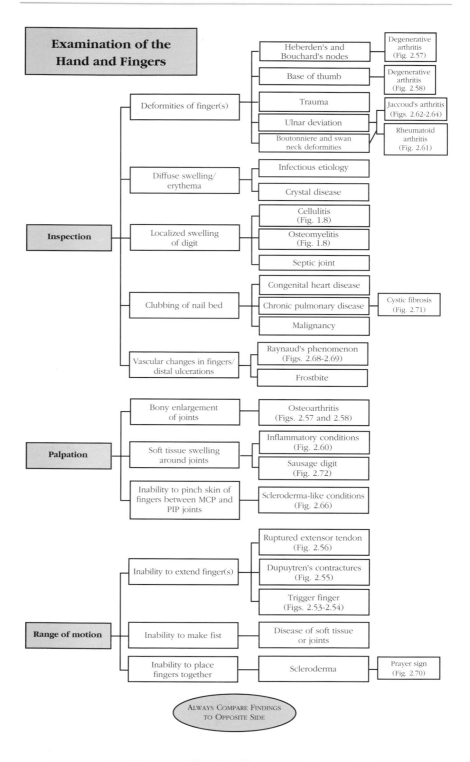

Examination of the Hand and Fingers

Inspection
- Deformities of finger(s)
  - Heberden's and Bouchard's nodes
    - Degenerative arthritis (Fig. 2.57)
  - Base of thumb
    - Degenerative arthritis (Fig. 2.58)
  - Trauma
  - Ulnar deviation
    - Jaccoud's arthritis (Figs. 2.62-2.64)
  - Boutonniere and swan neck deformities
    - Rheumatoid arthritis (Fig. 2.61)
- Diffuse swelling/erythema
  - Infectious etiology
  - Crystal disease
- Localized swelling of digit
  - Cellulitis (Fig. 1.8)
  - Osteomyelitis (Fig. 1.8)
  - Septic joint
- Clubbing of nail bed
  - Congenital heart disease
  - Chronic pulmonary disease
    - Cystic fibrosis (Fig. 2.71)
  - Malignancy
- Vascular changes in fingers/distal ulcerations
  - Raynaud's phenomenon (Figs. 2.68-2.69)
  - Frostbite

Palpation
- Bony enlargement of joints
  - Osteoarthritis (Figs. 2.57 and 2.58)
- Soft tissue swelling around joints
  - Inflammatory conditions (Fig. 2.60)
  - Sausage digit (Fig. 2.72)
- Inability to pinch skin of fingers between MCP and PIP joints
  - Scleroderma-like conditions (Fig. 2.66)

Range of motion
- Inability to extend finger(s)
  - Ruptured extensor tendon (Fig. 2.56)
  - Dupuytren's contractures (Fig. 2.55)
  - Trigger finger (Figs. 2.53-2.54)
- Inability to make fist
  - Disease of soft tissue or joints
- Inability to place fingers together
  - Scleroderma
    - Prayer sign (Fig. 2.70)

ALWAYS COMPARE FINDINGS TO OPPOSITE SIDE

FIGURES 2.53-2.54 **Trigger finger.** Patients with a trigger finger complain that their finger becomes stuck in a flexed position requiring them to use their opposite hand to release the finger. Palpation of the flexor tendon of the finger will usually demonstrate a nodule on the tendon that "catches" when it passes through the restraining pulley at the joint line.

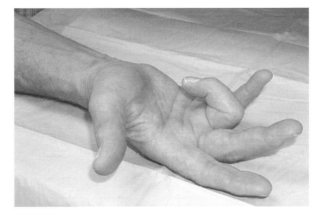

Figure 2.53 Trigger finger stuck in flexed position.

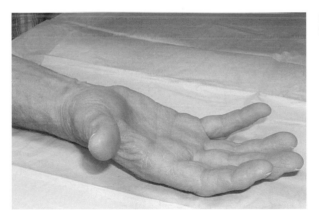

Figure 2.54 Trigger finger when released.

FIGURE 2.55 Dupuytren's contractures. The patient presents with a painless deformity of one or more fingers resulting in permanent flexion of the digits. The cause is generally unknown but may have a genetic component. The palmar fascia thickens and binds down the flexor tendons of the digits. The patient is therefore unable to extend his fingers. Dimpling of the skin in the palm of the hand may be observed.

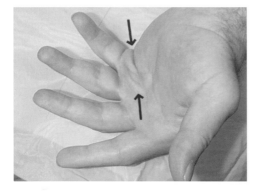

Figure 2.55 Dupuytren's contractures.

FIGURE 2.56 Extensor tendon rupture. An occasional patient may present with an inability to completely extend a digit but will have normal passive range of motion of the joint. In addition to checking for nerve damage, evaluation for rupture of the extensor tendon can be accomplished by palpating along the length of the tendon. Extensive synovial disease of the metacarpal phalangeal or wrist joints may result in tendon rupture.

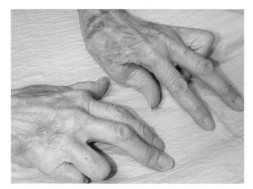

Figure 2.56 Lack of extension of 4th and 5th fingers.

FIGURES 2.57-2.60   **Finger joint deformities.** Bony or soft tissue involvement of the finger joints may result in significant deformity. A thorough joint examination of both upper and lower extremities will usually delineate the etiology. Bony swelling of the distal interphalangeal joint is consistent with Heberden's nodes, which are indicative of osteoarthritis. Bony enlargement of the first carpal metacarpal joint is pathognomonic for osteoarthritis and will result in the patient being unable to completely extend his thumb to the table when the hand is supinated. Bony swelling of the proximal interphalangeal joints is consistent with Bouchard's nodes. Synovitis of the interphalangeal joints such as seen in rheumatoid arthritis is described as a "boggy" or "spongy" feeling on bimanual palpation.

Figure 2.57 Bony enlargement in osteoarthritis.

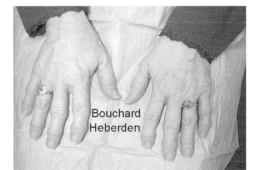

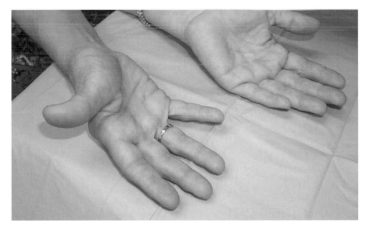

Figure 2.58 Thumb involvement in osteoarthritis.

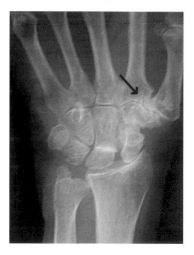

Figure 2.59 Radiographic evidence for degenerative arthritis of 1st carpal metacarpal joint.

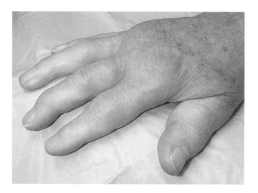

Figure 2.60 Synovitis of finger joints in rheumatoid arthritis.

FIGURES 2.61-2.64 **Ulnar deviation and Jaccoud's arthritis.** Ulnar deviation of the metacarpal phalangeal joints is a typical finding of rheumatoid arthritis due to subluxation of the joint with bony destruction. Jaccoud's arthritis is similar in appearance but is reducible by placing pressure on the metacarpal phalangeal joint.

Figure 2.61 Ulnar deviation with metacarpal subluxation.

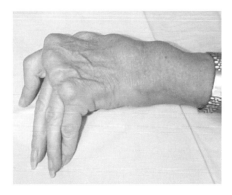

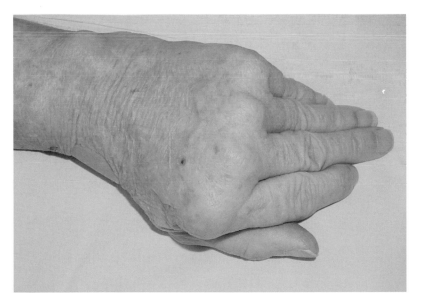

Figure 2.62 Jaccoud's arthritis in patient with systemic lupus erythematosus.

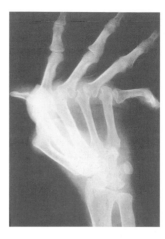

Figure 2.63 Radiograph of Jaccoud's arthritis showing subluxation.

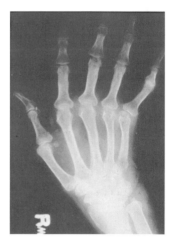

Figure 2.64 Radiograph of Jaccoud's arthritis with fingers straightened.

FIGURE 2.65 **Boutonniere/swan neck deformities.** Characteristically found in inflammatory arthritis such as rheumatoid disease, boutonniere and swan neck deformities are caused by synovitis destroying the tendon attachments around joints. The boutonniere deformity is flexion of the proximal interphalangeal joint with concomitant hyperextension of the distal joint. The opposite is seen in the swan neck deformity (hyperextension of the proximal and flexion of the distal interphalangeal joints).

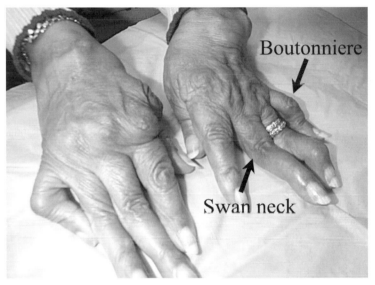

Figure 2.65 Hand deformities in rheumatoid arthritis.

FIGURES 2.66-2.67   **Pinch sign.** Tightness of the skin of the fingers (sclerodactyly) is a common finding in patients with scleroderma. In a normal individual, you can pinch the skin between the metacarpal phalangeal and proximal interphalangeal joint. In patients with scleroderma, the skin is too tight to pinch. In both normal and scleroderma patients, the skin between the proximal and distal interphalangeal joints cannot be pinched.

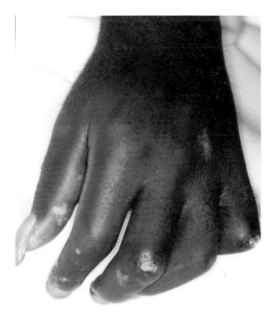

Figure 2.66   Tight skin of fingers.

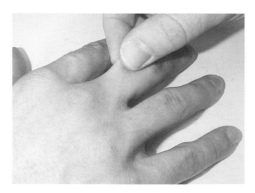

Figure 2.67   Individual with normal pinch sign.

FIGURES 2.68-2.69 **Raynaud's phenomenon.** Vasomotor instability with resultant white, cold, and painful digits is found in normal individuals and in some individuals with connective tissue diseases. The patient gives a history of blanching of one or more digits with exposure to cold and in stressful situations. Typically the blanching demarcates sharply at joint lines. The findings may be worsened by tobacco use. Nonhealing fingertip ulcers may be seen. The classic description of red, white, and blue color changes is not often mentioned by patients.

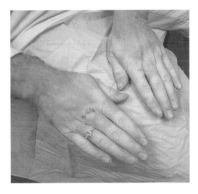

Figure 2.68 Raynaud's phenomenon (see Color Plate 8).

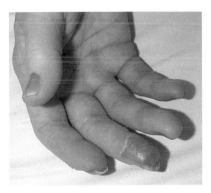

Figure 2.69 Nonhealing fingertip ulcer in patient with Raynaud's phenomenon (see Color Plate 9).

FIGURE 2.70 **Prayer sign.** The patient is asked to oppose the palmar surfaces of both hands. The inability to press the palms together suggests significant joint pathology. In patients with scleroderma, tightness of the skin prevents the patient from performing the test normally.

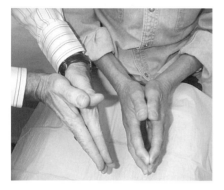

Figure 2.70 Prayer sign in patient with scleroderma (patient at right).

FIGURE 2.71 **Clubbing.** The angle between the nail bed and the long axis of the finger is normally more than 15°. Patients with a lesser angle have clubbed fingers, suggesting congenital heart disease, chronic pulmonary disease, or malignancy.

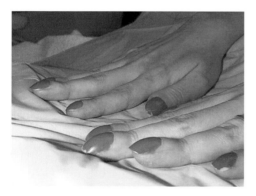

Figure 2.71 Clubbing in a patient with cystic fibrosis.

FIGURE **2.72** **Sausage digit.** Occasionally, swelling of the fingers results in diffuse enlargement of the digit(s), which is described as a sausage digit.

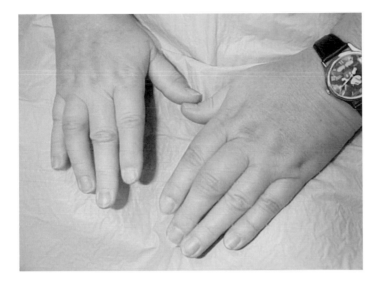

Figure 2.72 Sausage digit due to diffuse synovitis.

CHAPTER 3

SPINE AND GAIT

Spine

FIGURES 3.1-3.4 Cervical spine. Range of motion of the cervical spine consists of flexion to 45° and extension to 55°, lateral bending to approximately 40°, and rotation to 70°. The patient may demonstrate significant limitation of range of motion, which may be a manifestation of significant cervical vertebral body pathology or, more commonly, may be caused by muscle tightness. Arthritis is common in the cervical spine and results in decreased range of motion. The most common cause of pain in the neck is muscular; therefore examine carefully for muscle spasm or trigger points (particularly at the insertion of the cervical muscles in the occipital area).

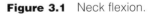

Figure 3.1 Neck flexion.

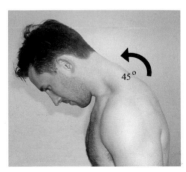

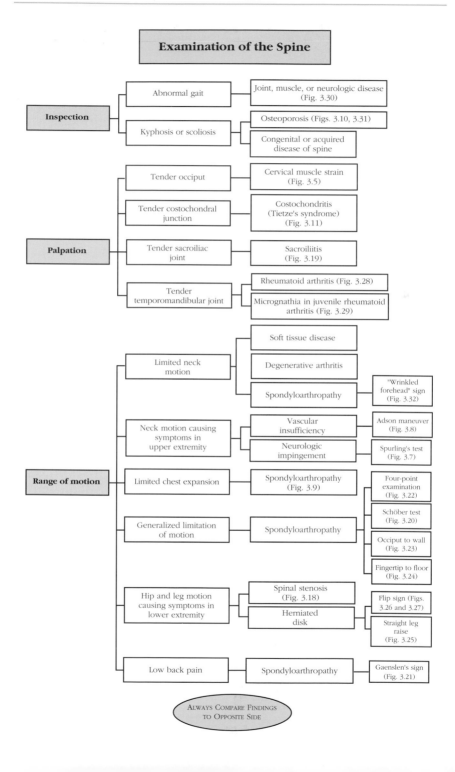

Examination of the Spine

Inspection
- Abnormal gait → Joint, muscle, or neurologic disease (Fig. 3.30)
- Kyphosis or scoliosis → Osteoporosis (Figs. 3.10, 3.31)
- Kyphosis or scoliosis → Congenital or acquired disease of spine

Palpation
- Tender occiput → Cervical muscle strain (Fig. 3.5)
- Tender costochondral junction → Costochondritis (Tietze's syndrome) (Fig. 3.11)
- Tender sacroiliac joint → Sacroiliitis (Fig. 3.19)
- Tender temporomandibular joint → Rheumatoid arthritis (Fig. 3.28)
- Tender temporomandibular joint → Micrognathia in juvenile rheumatoid arthritis (Fig. 3.29)

Range of motion
- Limited neck motion → Soft tissue disease
- Limited neck motion → Degenerative arthritis
- Limited neck motion → Spondyloarthropathy → "Wrinkled forehead" sign (Fig. 3.32)
- Neck motion causing symptoms in upper extremity → Vascular insufficiency → Adson maneuver (Fig. 3.8)
- Neck motion causing symptoms in upper extremity → Neurologic impingement → Spurling's test (Fig. 3.7)
- Limited chest expansion → Spondyloarthropathy (Fig. 3.9) → Four-point examination (Fig. 3.22)
- Generalized limitation of motion → Spondyloarthropathy → Schöber test (Fig. 3.20)
- Generalized limitation of motion → Spondyloarthropathy → Occiput to wall (Fig. 3.23)
- Generalized limitation of motion → Spondyloarthropathy → Fingertip to floor (Fig. 3.24)
- Hip and leg motion causing symptoms in lower extremity → Spinal stenosis (Fig. 3.18) → Flip sign (Figs. 3.26 and 3.27)
- Hip and leg motion causing symptoms in lower extremity → Herniated disk → Straight leg raise (Fig. 3.25)
- Low back pain → Spondyloarthropathy → Gaenslen's sign (Fig. 3.21)

ALWAYS COMPARE FINDINGS TO OPPOSITE SIDE

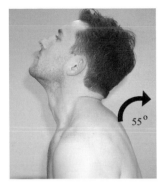

Figure 3.2 Neck extension.

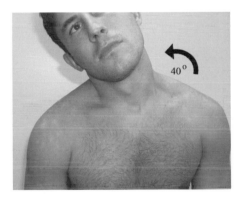

Figure 3.3 Lateral bending of neck.

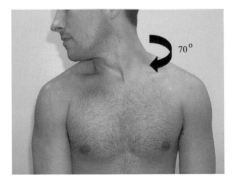

Figure 3.4 Lateral rotation of neck.

FIGURES 3.5-3.6   Occipital tenderness. Headache (particularly tension headache described as a tight band around the head) may be associated with cervical muscle spasm. Palpation of the insertion of the occipital muscles at the skull will duplicate the patient's pain in many cases. Pain radiating into the upper extremity may signify a neurologic process. Perform a complete neurologic examination on the upper extremity, checking reflexes, muscle strength, sensation, etc. Most acute radicular pain will resolve within several weeks to a few months and therefore should be treated conservatively. Progressive neurologic findings should be fully investigated with electromyography, nerve conduction studies, and magnetic resonance imaging or computed tomography where appropriate.

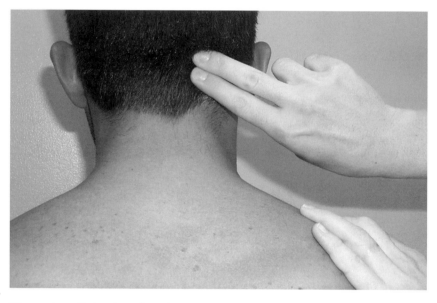

Figure 3.5   Palpation of occiput.

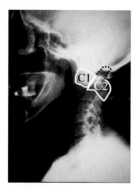

Figure 3.6   C1-C2 subluxation in a rheumatoid arthritis patient presenting with headache. Lateral radiograph of cervical spine with subluxation of C1 and C2 vertebral bodies outlined.

FIGURE 3.7   Spurling's test. Have the patient extend his neck while bending his head to the affected side. Patients with significant neurologic impingement will complain of radicular pain on that side.

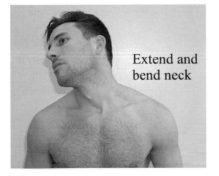

Figure 3.7   Spurling's test.

FIGURE 3.8   Adson maneuver for radial artery impingement. Palpate the radial artery at the wrist with the arm abducted to 90°. Obliteration of the pulse when the patient turns his head to the opposite side is a positive test.

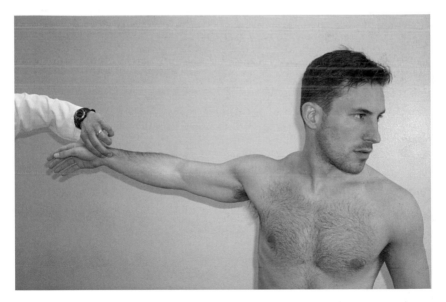

Figure 3.8   Adson maneuver.

Thoracic Spine

Range of motion of the thoracic spine is minimal. Likewise, findings on the normal musculoskeletal examination are minimal.

FIGURE 3.9   Chest expansion. Limitation of motion of the thoracolumbar spine may be found in spondyloarthropathies. In the thoracic area, limitation of chest expansion can be demonstrated by measuring the circumference of the chest at the nipple line in both full exhalation and inhalation. There should be 5 cm difference between the two measurements. If little difference between exhalation and inhalation is demonstrated, further investigation of the thoracic spine is appropriate.

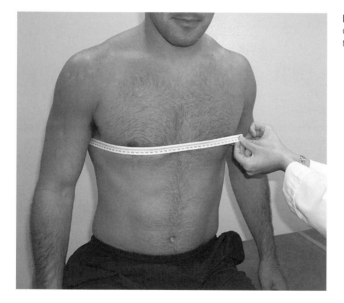

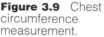

Figure 3.9 Chest circumference measurement.

Figure 3.10   **Back deformity.** Deformities of the back may indicate significant pathology. A gibbus deformity is classically associated with vertebral body collapse (from osteoporosis or pathologic replacement of bone). Exaggerated thoracic kyphosis is characteristic of osteoporosis (associated with significant loss of height). Tracing the spinous processes of each vertebral body and observing major deviation to either side can demonstrate scoliosis. Alternatively, have the patient bend at the waist and observe the two scapular areas. They should be at the same height unless scoliosis is present.

Figure 3.10 Severe kyphoscoliosis secondary to osteoporosis.

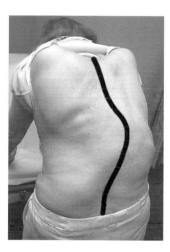

Figure 3.11   **Costochondritis (Tietze's syndome).** Tenderness over the costochondral junctions suggests costochondritis (Tietze's syndrome). Firm palpation over the affected area will duplicate the pain. Even though the costochondral junction is tender, one should still consider more serious causes of chest discomfort such as myocardial ischemia.

Figure 3.11 Palpation of costochondral junction.

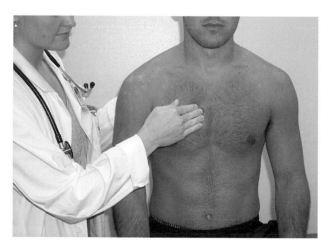

Lumbar Spine

Range of motion of the lumbar spine can be significantly decreased by many pathologic processes. The most common cause of decreased motion of the back is muscle involvement. A complete history and physical examination can help to delineate other etiologies of the patient's discomfort.

FIGURES 3.12-3.17   Normal flexion of the lumbar spine. Normal flexion of the lumbar spine is approximately 75° with hyperextension to 35°. Lateral bending and twisting are limited to 35° of motion.

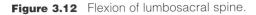

Figure 3.12   Flexion of lumbosacral spine.

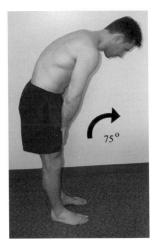

Figure 3.13   Extension of lumbosacral spine.

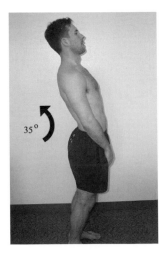

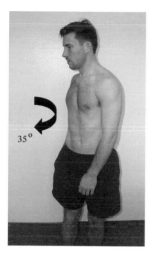

Figure 3.14 Twisting of lumbosacral spine to right.

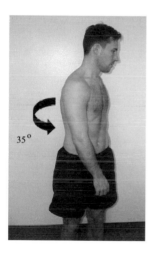

Figure 3.15 Twisting of lumbosacral spine to left.

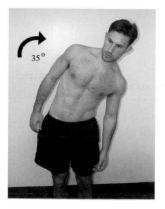

Figure 3.16 Bending of lumbosacral spine to left.

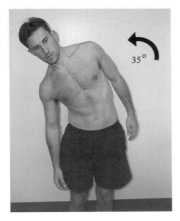

Figure 3.17 Bending of lumbosacral spine to right.

FIGURES 3.18-3.21   Back pain. The medical history is many times the best method to separate the various types of low back pain. Lumbar disk herniation usually begins acutely with pain aggravated by the Valsalva maneuver. Patients with spinal stenosis develop symptoms after variable amounts of physical activity. Pain will resolve when in a seated position. Sacroiliitis is characterized by morning stiffness in the low back lasting for more than 30 to 60 minutes. Sciatica causes pain that characteristically radiates from the ischial tuberosity down the back of the leg (not in a true dermatomal pattern) and may result from compression of the nerve by the piriform muscle.

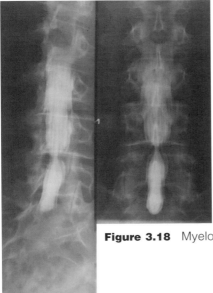

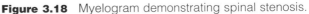

Figure 3.18 Myelogram demonstrating spinal stenosis.

FIGURE 3.19 **Sacroiliac tenderness.** Tenderness over the sacroiliac joint (located inferior to the posterior superior iliac spines) will be found in patients with active sacroiliitis. After the joint has fused, no tenderness will be noted but decreased range of motion of the lumbar spine will be demonstrated. Tenderness in the sacroiliac area is also noted in soft tissue pain syndromes such as fibromyalgia.

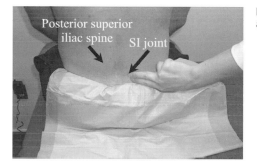

Figure 3.19 Palpation of sacroiliac joint.

FIGURE 3.20 **Schöber test.** This test is performed to determine if significant limitation of motion of the lumbar spine has occurred as a result of fusion of vertebral bodies. After locating the posterior superior iliac spines, place a mark over the spinal column between the two spines. Then measure up 10 cm and place another mark. Ask the patient to bend forward as much as possible. Normal individuals will increase the distance between the two marks by at least 3 to 5 cm. Fusion of the lumbar spine (either from surgical procedures or diseases such as ankylosing spondylitis) will result in a significant limitation of range of motion.

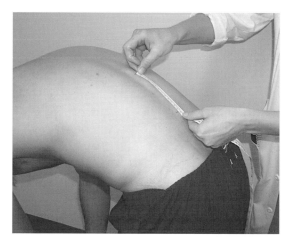

Figure 3.20 Measurement of spine with flexion.

FIGURE 3.21 **Gaenslen's sign.** Gaenslen's sign indicates sacroiliac disease. The patient places one buttock on the edge of the table and flexes that leg. The leg not on the table is allowed to drop to the floor, which stresses the sacroiliac joint. The patient with sacroilitis will complain of significant pain in the region of the sacroiliac joint.

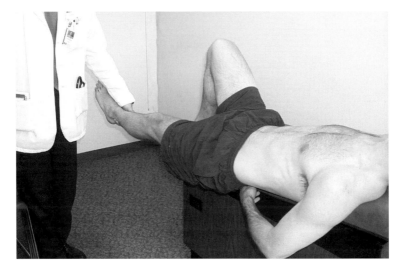

Figure 3.21 Gaenslen's sign.

FIGURE 3.22   Four-point examination. The four-point examination is an easy method for monitoring posture (particularly in a patient with spondyloarthropathy). The patient is asked to stand facing away from a wall or door while touching his occiput, thorax, buttocks, and heels against the surface. The examiner's hand should easily pass between the lumbar area and the wall. Failure to touch any of the four points to the wall suggests a problem with flexibility of the spinal column.

Figure 3.22   Four-point examination.

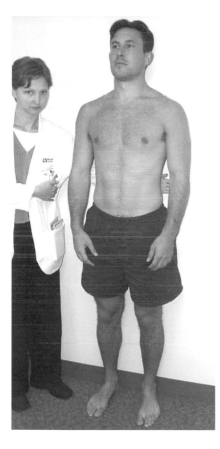

FIGURES 3.23-3.24 **Occiput to wall and fingertip to floor distance measurement.** The patient with spinal complaints will be unable to touch the wall or the floor when asked to perform this examination. Individuals in poor physical condition may have limitation of motion but do not demonstrate significant back pathology.

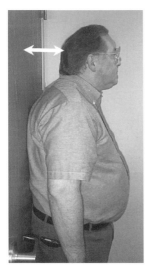

Figure 3.23 Occiput to wall.

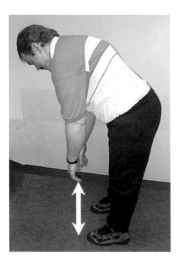

Figure 3.24 Fingertip to floor.

FIGURE 3.25   **Straight leg raising.** The patient is positioned supine on the examining table. The hip is flexed as the leg is raised. Patients with spinal stenosis, sciatica, lumbar disk herniation, or other disease processes may complain of pain radiating from the back down either or both legs. Stretching of nerve roots is presumed to be the cause of the pain. More specific neurologic testing, such as pain sensation, reflexes, and muscle strength testing, may help to further identify the disease process.

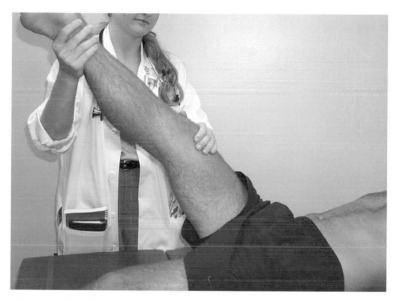

Figure 3.25   Straight leg raising examination.

FIGURES 3.26-3.27 **Flip sign.** With the patient sitting on the edge of the examining table, have him extend one knee. Patients with significant sciatic disease will flip back against the examining table with minimal extension of the knee. This correlates well with the straight leg raising examination.

Figure 3.26 Initiation of flip sign.

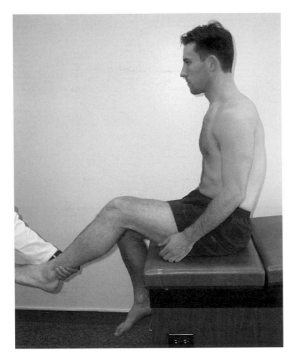

Figure 3.27 Positive flip sign.

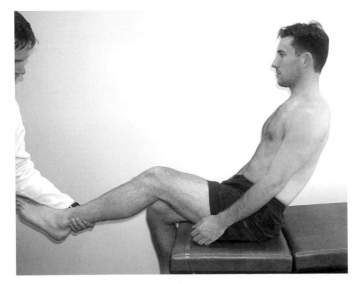

FIGURES 3.28-3.29 **Temporomandibular joint.** Involvement of the temporomandibular joint is most often secondary to trauma or a localized disease process. Perform a thorough external and oral examination. The temporomandibular joint is palpated anterior to the tragus while the patient opens and closes his mouth. If trauma can be excluded, pain over the joint suggests rheumatoid arthritis. Involvement of the growth plates in children with juvenile rheumatoid arthritis results in micrognathia.

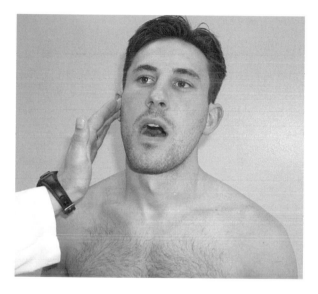

Figure 3.28 Palpation of temporomandibular joint.

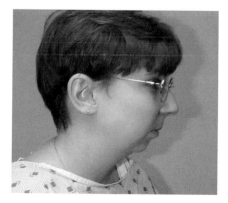

Figure 3.29 Micrognathia in a patient with juvenile rheumatoid arthritis.

Gait and Posture

FIGURE 3.30 Examination of gait. Observation of the patient's gait is a simple screen to determine if significant pathology of the spine or lower extremity is present. Observe the patient walking to determine if he favors one leg or the other. With pathology of one hip, the patient will limp with more time spent on the normal side than on the affected side. Patients with joint, muscular, or neurologic abnormalities demonstrate an uneven gait.

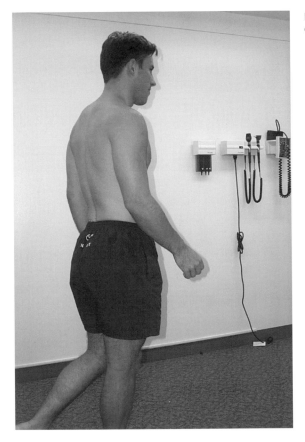

Figure 3.30 Examination of gait.

FIGURE 3.31 **Kyphoscoliosis.** An abnormality of posture may indicate that the patient has significant bony or muscular problems. Significant kyphoscoliosis indicates an underlying spinal abnormality (either muscular or bony) and suggests a need for appropriate radiography.

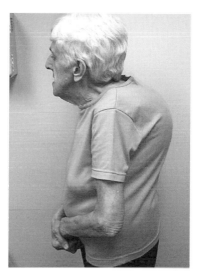

Figure 3.31 Severe kyphosis secondary to osteoporosis.

FIGURE 3.32   "Wrinkled forehead" sign. Patients with a spondyloarthropathy will have an abnormal posture as noted in the discussion of the lumbar spine (Figure 3.22). Patients with complete fusion of the spine will typically mover their entire spine *en bloc*. When asked to look to one side, the patient with a spondyloarthropathy will move his entire body rather than using a twisting motion as in a normal individual. If the patient is asked to look upward, he will demonstrate the "wrinkled forehead" sign.

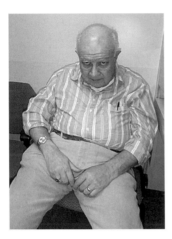

Figure 3.32   "Wrinkled forehead" sign in ankylosing spondylitis.

CHAPTER 4

LOWER EXTREMITIES

Disorders of the lower extremity are common and include many rheumatologic and soft tissue problems. A thorough examination of both extremities as well as the back is necessary. Abnormalities of either the joints or soft tissues may require further examination by a specialist.

Leg Length

FIGURE 4.1 **Leg length examination.** The leg length is measured from the anterior superior iliac spine to the medial malleolus. Comparison to the opposite side is important. A difference in length of less than 1 cm is expected.

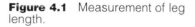

Figure 4.1 Measurement of leg length.

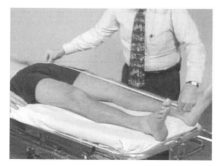

Hip

Figures 4.2-4.9 Hip. The hip is a ball-and-socket joint with six different movements. Flexion to 120° is normal. Hyperextension to 30° is demonstrated by having the patient lie prone on the table and extend his leg. Internal and external rotations are checked with the patient's hip and knee flexed. Normal range of motion is 40 to 45° for both movements. Rotation of the hip can also be examined by moving the ankle of the straight leg internally and externally. An individual with hip pathology will rotate the pelvis to protect the hip. Abduction is normally 45°, and adduction is approximately 30°. True hip pain is described as pain in the groin, whereas symptoms of trochanteric bursitis are lateral to the hip joint in the area of the greater trochanter.

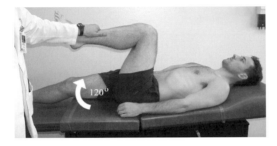

Figure 4.2 Hip flexion.

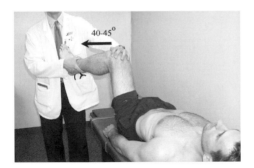

Figure 4.3 Internal rotation of hip with knee flexed.

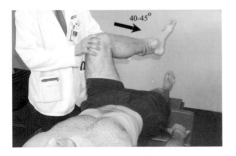

Figure 4.4 External rotation of hip with knee flexed.

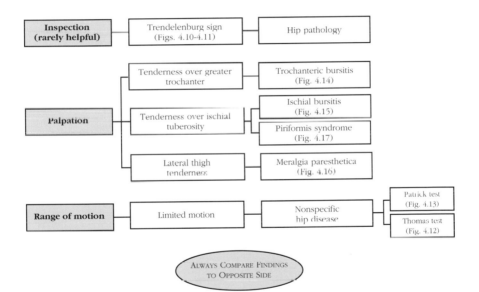

Examination of the Hip

Inspection (rarely helpful) — Trendelenburg sign (Figs. 4.10-4.11) — Hip pathology

Palpation —
- Tenderness over greater trochanter — Trochanteric bursitis (Fig. 4.14)
- Tenderness over ischial tuberosity — Ischial bursitis (Fig. 4.15) / Piriformis syndrome (Fig. 4.17)
- Lateral thigh tenderness — Meralgia paresthetica (Fig. 4.16)

Range of motion — Limited motion — Nonspecific hip disease — Patrick test (Fig. 4.13) / Thomas test (Fig. 4.12)

ALWAYS COMPARE FINDINGS TO OPPOSITE SIDE

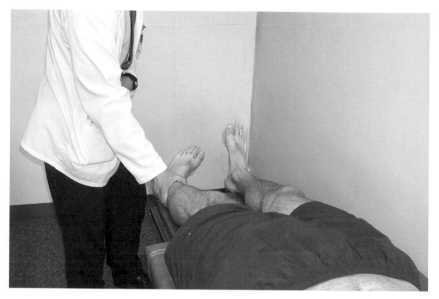

Figure 4-5   Internal rotation of hip with log roll.

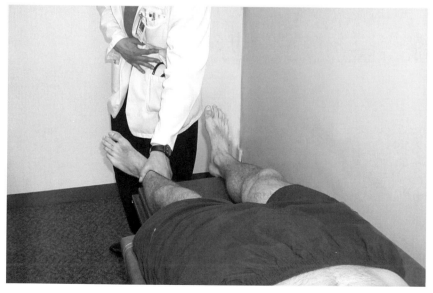

Figure 4.6   External rotation of hip with log roll.

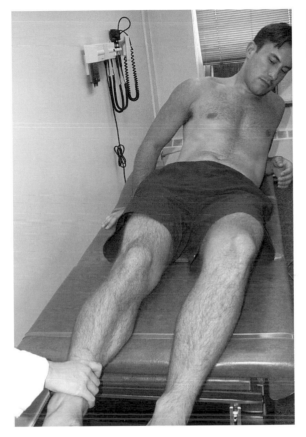

Figure 4.7 Internal rotation. Note that the patient is rotating his pelvis to protect his hip from pain.

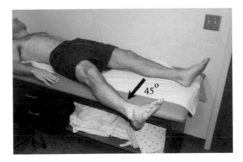

Figure 4.8 Abduction of the hip.

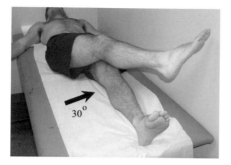

Figure 4.9 Adduction of the hip.

FIGURES 4.10-4.11   **Trendelenburg sign.** Ask the patient to stand on one leg. Normally, the pelvis on the opposite side will tilt up. If the iliac crest drops on the opposite side, suspect significant hip disease on the weight-bearing side.

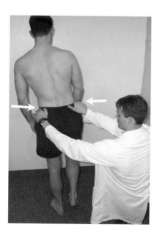

Figure 4.10 Trendelenburg sign: normal (weight on left leg).

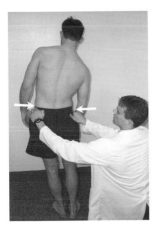

Figure 4.11   Trendelenburg sign: abnormal (weight on left leg).

FIGURE 4.12   **Thomas test.** The Thomas test is used to test for flexion contracture of the hip. The patient is asked to flex one hip to the chest. In normal individuals, the opposite leg will remain flat on the table. Patients with significant hip pathology will begin to flex the noninvolved hip to compensate.

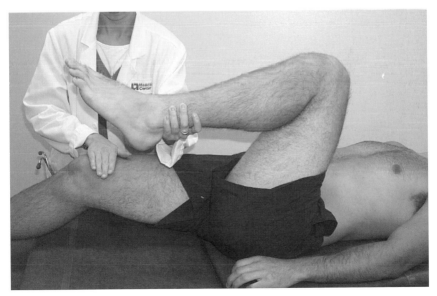

Figure 4.12   Thomas test.

FIGURE 4.13 Patrick test. Instruct the patient to place the lateral aspect of his foot on the opposite knee. The flexed leg is then moved toward the examining table. Approximately 45° of motion is expected. Hip pathology will limit the patient's ability to perform this test.

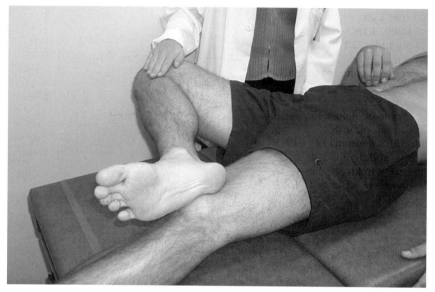

Figure 4.13 Patrick test.

Bursitis

FIGURE **4.14   Trochanteric bursitis.** Inflammation of the trochanteric bursa is a common cause of "hip" pain. The patient complains of a "burning" sensation and has difficulty sleeping on the affected side. Palpation over the area will duplicate the patient's symptoms. Pain may be worse with external rotation and abduction.

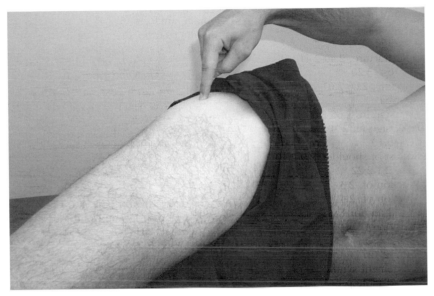

Figure 4.14   Location of trochanteric bursa.

FIGURE 4.15 **Ischial bursitis.** Tenderness over the ischial tuberosity is found in ischial bursitis (weaver's bottom). This condition is often found in thin individuals who sit for prolonged periods on hard surfaces. Direct palpation will demonstrate tenderness.

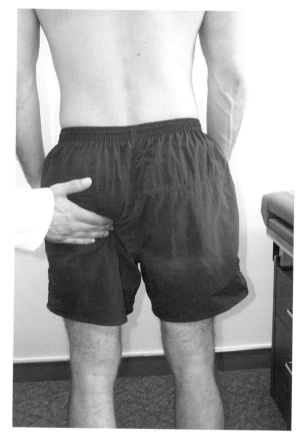

Figure 4.15 Palpation of ischial bursa.

FIGURE 4.16 **Meralgia paresthetica.** Compression of the lateral femoral cutaneous nerve medial to the anterior superior iliac spine as it leaves the pelvis causes lateral leg burning and pain. Tenderness may be elicited over the anterolateral thigh.

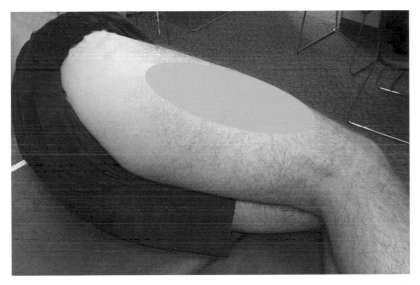

Figure 4.16 Approximate area of lateral femoral cutaneous nerve distribution.

FIGURE 4.17 **Piriformis syndrome.** This ill-defined syndrome results in pain over the buttocks and radiation into the leg along the sciatic nerve. Prolonged sitting may aggravate the condition. Rectal or vaginal examination demonstrates tenderness of the piriformis muscle.

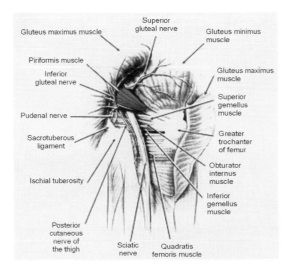

Figure 4.17 Gross anatomy of the piriformis muscle.

Knee

FIGURES 4.18-4.19   **Knee.** The knee is often the cause of significant disability for individuals with joint or soft tissue problems. Careful examination is necessary to delineate the etiology of the patient's problems. The normal knee flexes to 130° and hyperextends to –15°. A varus or valgus deformity of the knee is often the first physical abnormality identified and may signify underlying pathology. After acute trauma, many of the listed tests are difficult to perform and interpret.

Figure 4.18   Knee flexion.

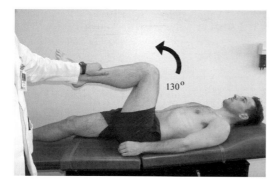

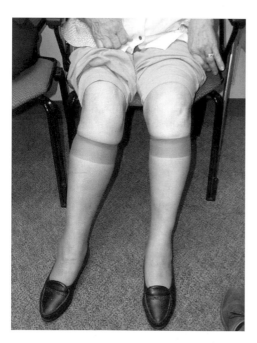

Figure 4.19   Valgus deformity of right knee.

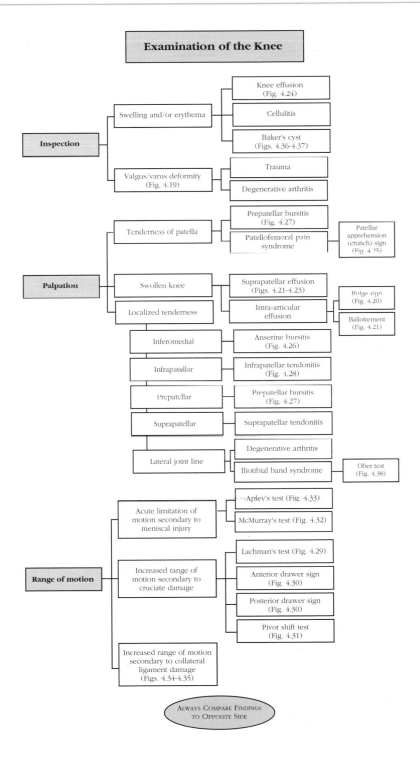

Examination of the Knee

Inspection
- Swelling and/or erythema
  - Knee effusion (Fig. 4.24)
  - Cellulitis
  - Baker's cyst (Figs. 4.36-4.37)
- Valgus/varus deformity (Fig. 4.19)
  - Trauma
  - Degenerative arthritis

Palpation
- Tenderness of patella
  - Prepatellar bursitis (Fig. 4.27)
  - Patellofemoral pain syndrome — Patellar apprehension (crunch) sign (Fig. 4.25)
- Swollen knee
  - Suprapatellar effusion (Figs. 4.21-4.23) — Bulge sign (Fig. 4.20)
  - Intra-articular effusion — Ballottement (Fig. 4.21)
- Localized tenderness
  - Inferomedial — Anserine bursitis (Fig. 4.26)
  - Infrapatellar — Infrapatellar tendonitis (Fig. 4.28)
  - Prepatellar — Prepatellar bursitis (Fig. 4.27)
  - Suprapatellar — Suprapatellar tendonitis
  - Lateral joint line
    - Degenerative arthritis
    - Iliotibial band syndrome — Ober test (Fig. 4.38)

Range of motion
- Acute limitation of motion secondary to meniscal injury
  - Apley's test (Fig. 4.33)
  - McMurray's test (Fig. 4.32)
- Increased range of motion secondary to cruciate damage
  - Lachman's test (Fig. 4.29)
  - Anterior drawer sign (Fig. 4.30)
  - Posterior drawer sign (Fig. 4.30)
  - Pivot shift test (Fig. 4.31)
- Increased range of motion secondary to collateral ligament damage (Figs. 4.34-4.35)

ALWAYS COMPARE FINDINGS TO OPPOSITE SIDE

FIGURE 4.20 Bulge sign. Normally the knee joint contains less than 5 mL of synovial fluid. The bulge sign can be used to determine if excessive fluid is present. The patient is placed supine on the examining table. It is very important that the patient is relaxed. Fluid, if present, is gradually milked from one side of the knee to the opposite (either medial to lateral or lateral to medial). Then gently press on the side to which the fluid was milked and observe the area between the patella and femur on the opposite side from where pressure has been placed. The development of a "bulge" indicates the presence of fluid. Be aware that transmission of the wave through fat may simulate a positive bulge sign.

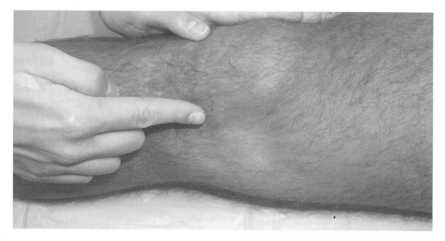

Figure 4.20 Identification of area where "bulge" will be seen.

FIGURE 4.21 Ballottement. An alternative method of determining if an increase in synovial fluid is present is ballottement. With the patient relaxed in the supine position, gently force the patella against the femur. Quickly release the patella and feel for the quick rebound of the patella, similar to a fluid wave in the abdomen.

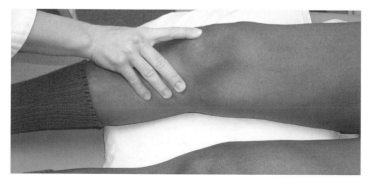

Figure 4.21 Ballottement test.

FIGURES 4.22-4.24   **Suprapatellar effusion.** The presence of a suprapatellar effusion can be suggested by forcing any fluid to move toward the knee with firm pressure directed toward the patella. If fluid is present, your hand will be stopped from reaching the area of the patella by the effusion.

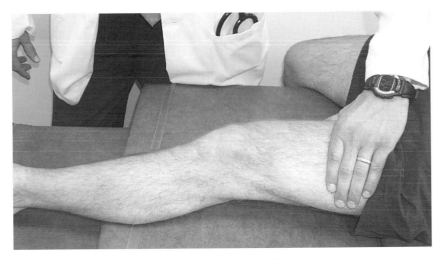

Figure 4.22   Initiation of pressure towards patella.

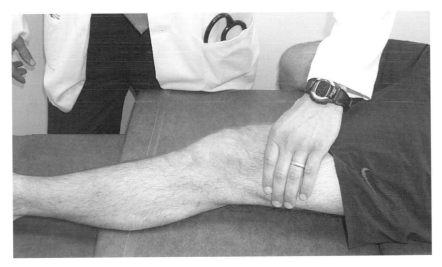

Figure 4.23   Hand position at end of procedure.

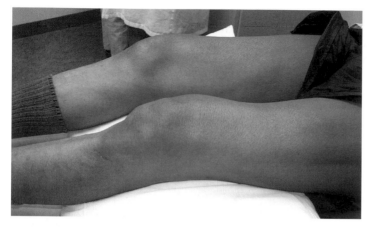

Figure 4.24 Large bilateral effusions.

FIGURE 4.25 Patellar apprehension (crunch) sign. Pain in the knee (particularly when going up or down stairs) is characteristic of the patellofemoral pain syndrome or chondromalacia patella. Patients will describe pain in the knee when the knee is actively extended while downward pressure is placed on the patella.

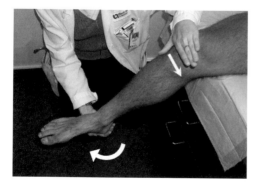

Figure 4.25 Patellar apprehension (crunch) sign.

Bursitis/Tendonitis

Bursitis and tendonitis are common causes of knee pain. Patients usually do not locate their pain directly over the involved area so careful palpation of the appropriate areas of the knee is necessary.

FIGURE 4.26 **Anserine bursitis.** One of the most common causes of knee pain is anserine bursitis. The bursa is located at the medial insertion of the hamstring muscles (semimembranosus, semitendinosus, and sartorius) on the proximal tibia. Tenderness in this location is often the cause of chronic knee pain.

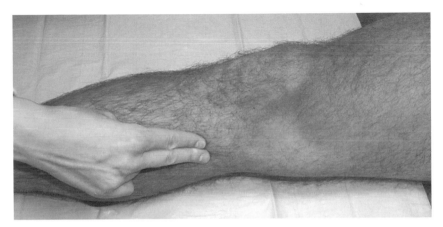

Figure 4.26 Palpation of the anserine bursa.

FIGURE 4.27 **Prepatellar bursitis.** Prepatellar bursitis, similar to olecranon bursitis in the elbow, presents with swelling, pain, and other signs of inflammation anterior to the patella. Care must be taken to differentiate this condition from the findings of a septic joint. In general, patients with prepatellar bursitis will have findings limited to the anterior knee, whereas an individual with a septic joint will demonstrate abnormalities circumferentially around the joint.

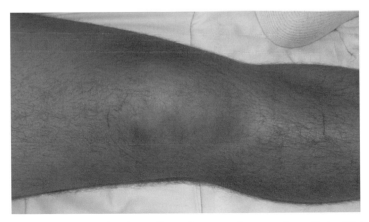

Figure 4.27 Minimal swelling of prepatellar area (see Color Plate 10).

FIGURE 4.28   Quadriceps/infrapatellar tendonitis. Pain over the insertion of the quadriceps tendon on the patella or tenderness of the insertion of the patellar tendon into the tibia is characteristically found. Pain in the area of the tibial insertion of the tendon is also seen in Osgood-Schlatter disease (classically found in teenagers).

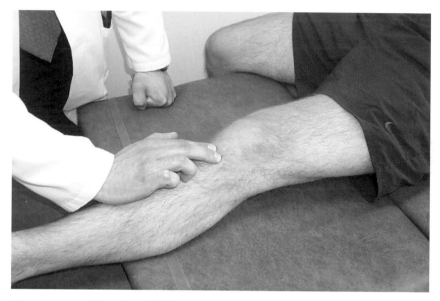

Figure 4.28   Palpation of infrapatellar area.

Cruciate Damage

FIGURE 4.29   Lachman's test. The best test for cruciate damage is Lachman's test. With the patient's knee flexed 20 to 30°, grasp the upper leg with one hand and the lower leg with the opposite hand. Displace one hand posteriorly while pulling anteriorly with the other hand. Increased movement in one direction suggests damage to the cruciate ligament. This test is difficult to perform if the examiner has small hands or the patient's leg is large. In that situation, the drawer sign test (Figure 4.30) should be performed.

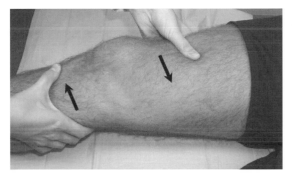

Figure 4.29 Lachman's test.

FIGURE 4.30 **Anterior/posterior drawer sign test.** Damage to the ante rior and posterior cruciate ligaments is documented by this test. The patient is placed supine on the table with the knee flexed. Sit on the patient's foot to stabilize the leg. Grasp the lower leg at the upper portion of the tibia while alternately pulling anteriorly and pushing posteriorly. An increase in motion in either of these motions suggests cruciate damage. Compare with the opposite side to determine if an abnormality is present.

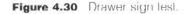

Figure 4.30 Drawer sign test.

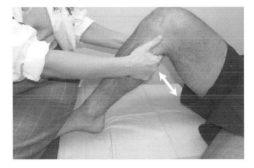

FIGURE 4.31   Pivot shift test. The pivot shift test helps check for anterior cruciate tear. The leg is fully extended and internally rotated. Flex the knee while applying a valgus force to the knee. At about 30°, a "jump" occurs as the tibia returns to its normal position on the femur.

Figure 4.31 Pivot shift test.

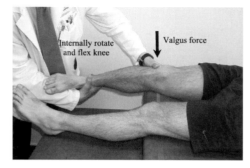

Meniscal Examination

FIGURE 4.32   McMurray's test. McMurray's test is done to check for medial or collateral meniscal tears. The patient is placed in the supine position with the knee fully flexed. Grasp the lower leg and extend the knee with external or internal rotation. Joint line pain or an audible click or locking sensation suggests meniscal damage. This test is not specific and must be confirmed with MRI or arthrography.

Figure 4.32 McMurray's test.

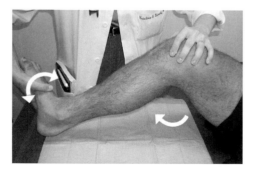

FIGURE 4.33 **Apley's test.** Apley's test also checks for meniscal damage. The patient is placed in the prone position with the knee flexed to 90°. Downward pressure is applied to the foot while the leg is internally and externally rotated. As with McMurray's test (Figure 4.32), any audible click, locking sensation, or pain in the joint line suggests meniscal pathology.

Figure 4.33 Apley's test.

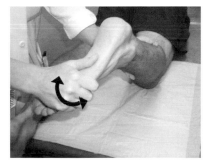

FIGURES 4.34-4.35 **Collateral ligament testing.** Have the supine patient flex his knee to 30°. To check for lateral ligament insufficiency, place one hand on the medial aspect of the joint while holding the ankle firmly in place. Varus pressure (outward) is placed on the medial joint area while firmly fixing the ankle in position. Excessive movement should be compared with the movement of the other knee to determine if this is a significant problem or is a normal finding for the individual being examined. The medial collateral ligament is similarly examined. Valgus pressure (toward the midline) at the joint line should not result in significant movement of the joint. If laxity in the joint is noted, check the other knee to see if a difference in movement between the two joints is detected. This is suggestive of medial collateral ligament insufficiency.

Figure 4.34 Testing the lateral collateral ligament.

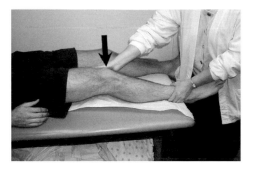

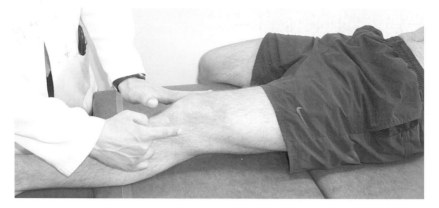

Figure 4.35 Testing the medial collateral ligament.

Figures 4.36-4.37 **Baker's cyst.** A Baker's cyst is an outpoaching of the synovium of the knee into the popliteal area. It is commonly found in both degenerative and rheumatoid arthritis as well as trauma. The patient is examined in a standing position. The popliteal area is palpated for any fullness or cyst-like structure. It is often difficult to definitively identify a cyst if there is significant adipose tissue in the knee. Rupture of a Baker's cyst will cause acute calf pain and swelling; the patient may not have noticed popliteal swelling before the rupture. Measurement of the calf circumference at a fixed point below the tibial tubercle can be compared with that of the opposite side. Because it is extremely difficult to differentiate a Baker's cyst from a deep venous thrombosis, appropriate Doppler ultrasonography, arthrography, or MRI should be performed.

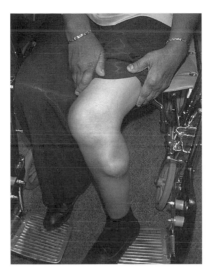

Figure 4.36 Unusual lateral Baker's cyst.

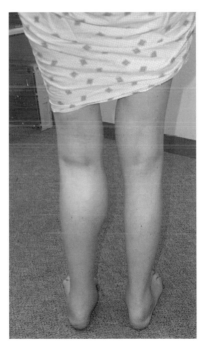

Figure 4.37 Swollen left calf from ruptured Baker's cyst.

FIGURE 4.38 **Ober test.** The Ober test is used to diagnosis iliotibial band syndrome. The patient is positioned on the nonaffected side with the hip flexed. The upper leg is held in abduction by the examiner, with the knee flexed to 90°. When the leg is released, the patient with iliotibial band syndrome will not be able to adduct the leg. Pain over the distal lateral thigh or lateral knee will be reported.

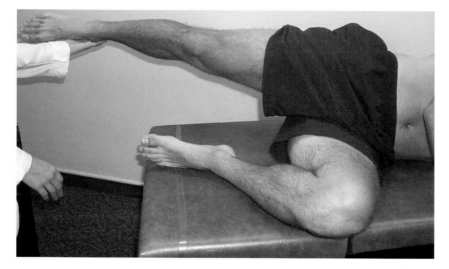

Figure 4.38 Ober test.

Ankle

FIGURES 4.39-4.40 **Ankle.** Soft tissue and joint disease of the ankle may cause the patient to have considerable difficulty with ambulation. A thorough examination is required to make the appropriate diagnosis and initiate therapy. The subtalar joint allows 30° of inversion and 20° of eversion. Ten to 20° of abduction and adduction are normally present. Dorsiflexion of the ankle is limited to 20°, plantar flexion to 45°.

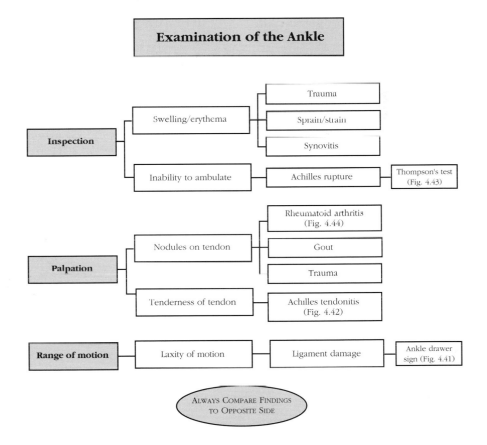

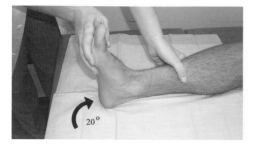

Figure 4.39 Dorsiflexion of ankle.

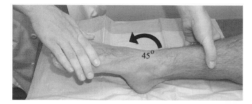

Figure 4.40 Plantar flexion of ankle.

FIGURE 4.41 Ankle drawer sign. The ankle drawer sign can check weakness of the ligaments of the ankle. With the patient sitting, place posterior pressure on the distal tibia while pulling the heel forward. Unusual laxity of the joint should be checked against the other side.

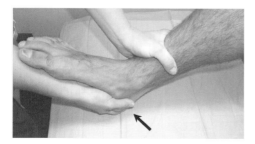

Figure 4.41 Ankle drawer sign.

FIGURE 4.42 **Achilles tendonitis.** Achilles tendonitis, sometimes known as lover's heel, causes inflammatory changes in the insertion of the Achilles tendon at the calcaneus. Swelling, redness, and tenderness are present. Reactive arthritis and gonococcal arthritis are two common causes of this condition. Sever's disease is a strain at the insertion of the Achilles tendon into the calcaneus (calcaneal apophysitis), which is similar in etiology to Osgood-Schlatter disease in the knee.

Figure 4.42 Swelling of ankle secondary to reactive arthritis.

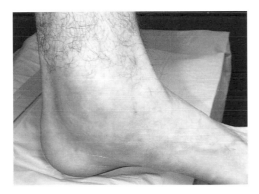

FIGURE 4.43 **Thompson's test for Achilles tendon rupture.** A complete tear of the Achilles tendon is a serious problem that requires immediate orthopedic consultation. Ask the patient to kneel on a chair. Tightly grasp the calf muscles while pressing upward to the knee. This procedure should result in plantar flexion of the foot if the Achilles tendon is intact.

Figure 4.43 Thompson's test.

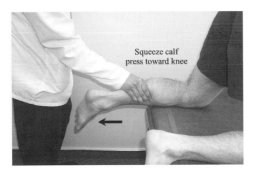

Squeeze calf
press toward knee

FIGURE 4.44   Achilles nodules. Nodular growths on the Achilles tendon may be secondary to trauma or represent gouty tophi or rheumatoid nodules.

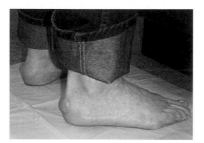

Figure 4.44 Rheumatoid nodules on Achilles tendon.

Sprains/Strains

Ankle sprains and strains are common injuries due to forced inversion or eversion of the foot. A *strain* results from increased laxity of the ligaments of the ankle. A *sprain* indicates partial or complete tear of the ligaments. Varus and valgus stress on the ankle may demonstrate increased movement on the affected side.

FIGURE 4.45   Principal ligaments of the ankle. Damage to any of the principal ligaments of the ankle can result in the patient having significant pain and disability. Any apparent laxity of the ankle during the examination should be compared to the opposite side.

Figure 4.45 Ligaments of the ankle.

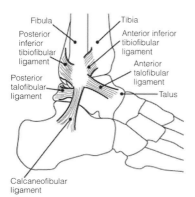

Fibula
Posterior inferior tibiofibular ligament
Posterior talofibular ligament
Calcaneofibular ligament
Tibia
Anterior inferior tibiofibular ligament
Anterior talofibular ligament
Talus

Foot and Toes

FIGURES 4.46-4.47   **Dactylitis.** Observation and palpation of the foot and toes will be adequate to identify various disease processes that may cause disability. Palpation of the metatarsal phalangeal (MTP) joints is done with the thumb on one side of the joint pressing against a finger on the other side. Pain reproduced with this examination is suggestive of synovial involvement.

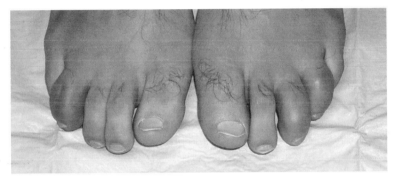

Figure 4.46   Dactylitis (inflammation) of toes in reactive arthritis (see Color Plate 11).

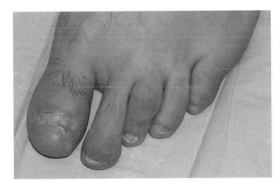

Figure 4.47   Dactylitis (inflammation) in psoriatic arthritis (see Color Plate 12).

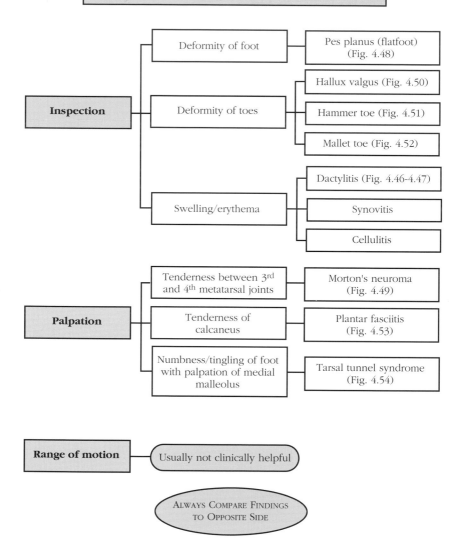

Examination of the Foot and Toes

Inspection

Deformity of foot → Pes planus (flatfoot) (Fig. 4.48)

Deformity of toes → Hallux valgus (Fig. 4.50)
Hammer toe (Fig. 4.51)
Mallet toe (Fig. 4.52)

Swelling/erythema → Dactylitis (Fig. 4.46-4.47)
Synovitis
Cellulitis

Palpation

Tenderness between 3rd and 4th metatarsal joints → Morton's neuroma (Fig. 4.49)

Tenderness of calcaneus → Plantar fasciitis (Fig. 4.53)

Numbness/tingling of foot with palpation of medial malleolus → Tarsal tunnel syndrome (Fig. 4.54)

Range of motion — Usually not clinically helpful

ALWAYS COMPARE FINDINGS TO OPPOSITE SIDE

FIGURE 4.48 **Common foot deformities.** Common deformities of the foot include pes valgus (out-toeing), pes varus (in-toeing), and pes planus (flatfoot). These abnormalities can be identified by observing the patient ambulate.

Figure 4.48 Pes planus (flatfoot).

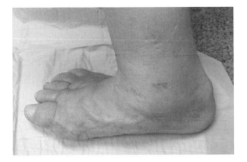

FIGURE 4.49 **Morton's neuroma.** Palpation of the area between the 3rd and 4th metatarsal head may reveal a pea-sized mass. Morton's neuroma consists of fibrotic nerve tissue that causes plantar pain and occasional numbness in the distal toes.

Figure 4.49 Palpation of Morton's neuroma.

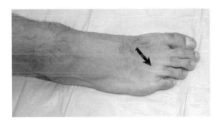

FIGURES 4.50-4.52 Toe deformities. Many deformities of the toes have been described. They are usually secondary to ill-fitting shoes, trauma, or underlying arthritis. Simple observation can usually identify the abnormality.

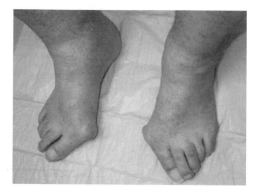

Figure 4.50 Hallux valgus: lateral deviation of the great toe. There is strong familial tendency and female predominance for hallux valgus.

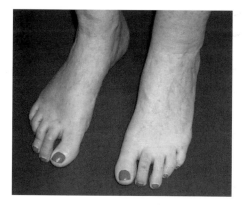

Figure 4.51 Hammer toe: flexion of the proximal interphalangeal joints with extension of the distal joint. Shown here is hammer toe deformity of right third toe.

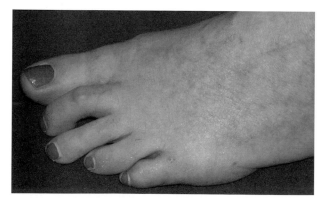

Figure 4.52 Mallet toe: flexion of the distal interphalangeal joint. Shown here is mallet toe deformity of second toe.

FIGURE 4.53 **Plantar fasciitis.** Severe pain with early morning ambulation is characteristic of plantar fasciitis. Firm palpation over the insertion of the plantar fascia onto the calcaneus will duplicate the patient's symptoms.

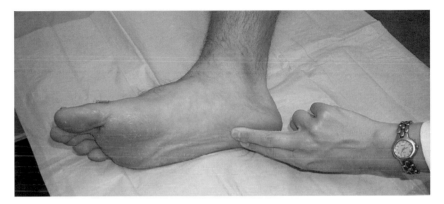

Figure 4.53 Palpation for plantar fasciitis.

FIGURE 4.54 **Tarsal tunnel syndrome.** Compression of the posterior tibial nerve below the medial malleolus results in numbness, tingling, and dysesthesia of the sole of the foot. Palpate the area to determine if irritation of the nerve duplicates the patient's complaints.

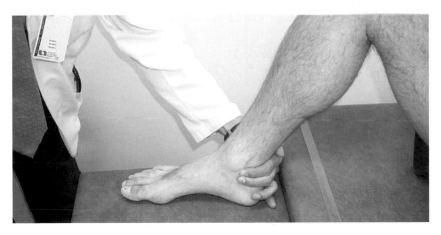

Figure 4.54 Palpation of posterior tibial nerve.

Fibromyalgia

FIGURES 4.55-4.57 **Fibromyalgia.** Patients who present with chronic pain, particularly in and around joints, should be carefully examined to determine if joint pathology can be demonstrated. Many of these individuals may have fibromyalgia, a chronic noninflammatory process. Patients will have multiple trigger points on physical examination. Many of these trigger points have already been discussed: occipital insertion of cervical musculature (Figure 3.5), costochondral junction (Figure 3.11), lateral epicondyle (Figures 2.31 and 2.32), greater trochanteric bursa (Figure 4.14), and anserine bursa (Figure 4.26). A patient with tenderness to palpation over at least 11 of 18 trigger points can be said to have fibromyalgia (Table 4.1).

Table 4.1 Eighteen Trigger Points of Fibromyalgia (All Found Symmetrically)

Occiput	Figure 3.5
Mid-trapezius	Figure 4.56
Mid-rhomboid	Figure 4.55
Costochondral junction	Figure 3.11
Subdeltoid	Figure 4.57
Lateral epicondyle	Figures 2.31-2.32
Sacroiliac	Figure 3.19
Greater trochanteric bursa	Figure 4.14
Anserine bursa	Figure 4.26

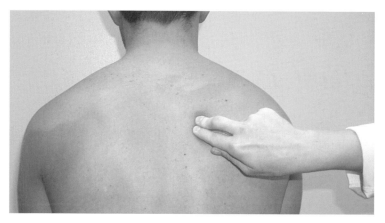

Figure 4.55 Palpation of the mid-rhomboid area.

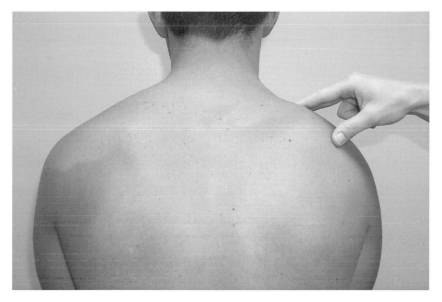

Figure 4.56 Palpation of the trapezius muscle.

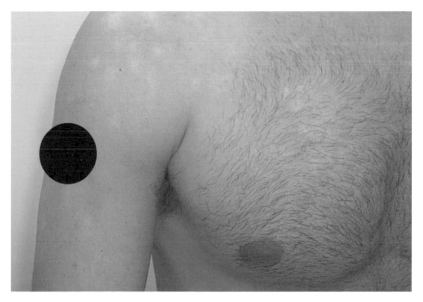

Figure 4.57 Location of subdeltoid trigger point.

INDEX

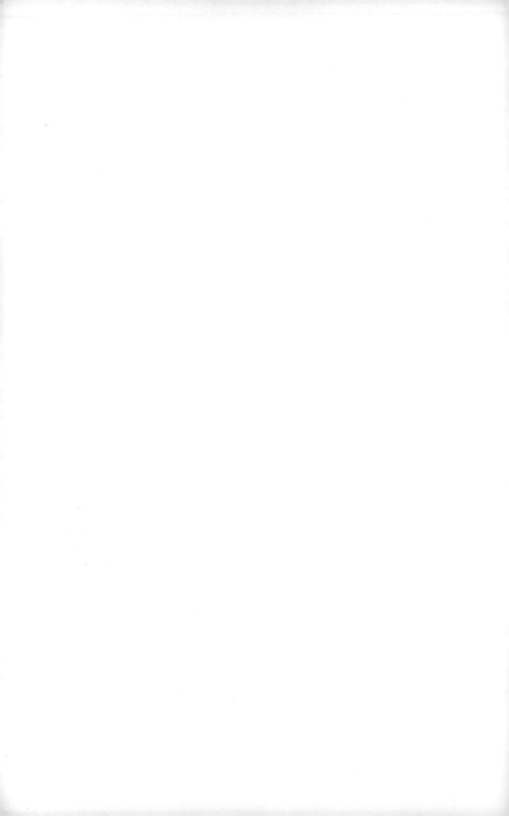

Color Plates

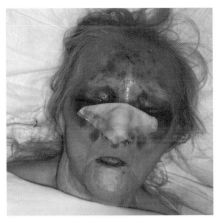

Plate 1 Patient with ecchmymoses secondary to head trauma.

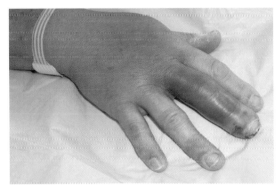

Plate 2 Osteomyelitis with cellulitis in third digit.

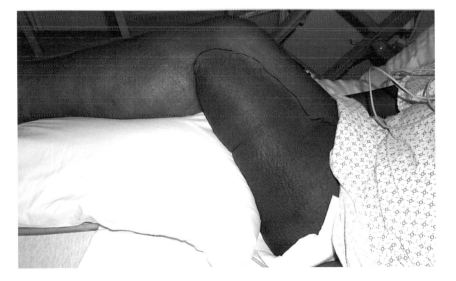

Plate 3 Cellulitis of proximal thigh.

Color Plates

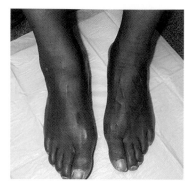

Plate 4 Inflammation of right ankle.

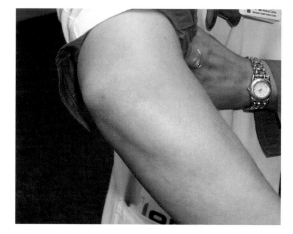

Plate 5 Cellulitis of elbow.

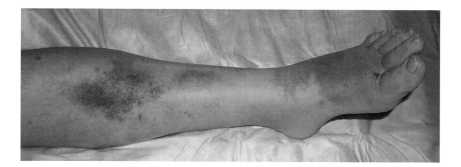

Plate 6 Cellulitis of lower leg.

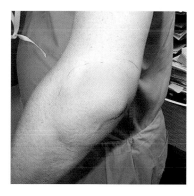

Plate 7 Inflamed olecranon bursa.

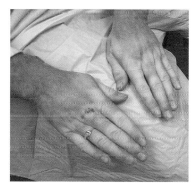

Plate 8 Raynaud's phenomenon.

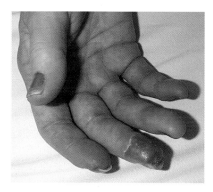

Plate 9 Nonhealing fingertip ulcer in patient with Raynaud's phenomenon.

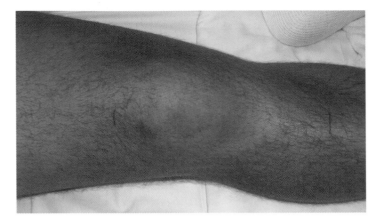

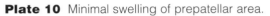

Plate 10 Minimal swelling of prepatellar area.

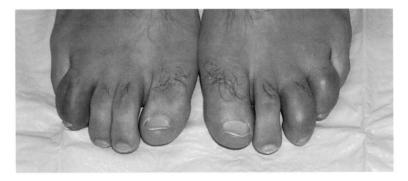

Plate 11 Dactylitis (inflammation) of toes in reactive arthritis.

Plate 12 Dactylitis (inflammation) in psoriatic arthritis.

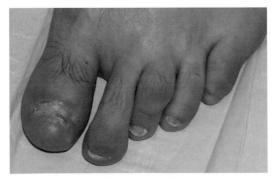